Wound Healing
and Wound Infection

Wound Healing and Wound Infection
Theory and Surgical Practice

Edited by

Thomas K. Hunt, M.D.

Professor of Surgery and Ambulatory and Community Medicine
Department of Surgery, School of Medicine
University of California, San Francisco, California

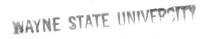

APPLETON-CENTURY-CROFTS/New York

80 81 82 83 84 10 9 8 7 6 5 4 3 2 1

Prentice-Hall International, Inc., London
Prentice-Hall of Australia, Pty. Ltd., Sydney
Prentice-Hall of India Private Limited, New Delhi
Prentice-Hall of Japan, Inc., Tokyo
Prentice-Hall of Southeast Asia (Pte.) Ltd., Singapore
Whitehall Books Ltd., Wellington, New Zealand

Library of Congress Cataloging in Publication Data

Main entry under title:

Wound healing and wound infection.

    Papers presented at a symposium held in San
Francisco in 1977 which was sponsored by the Minnesota
Mining and Manufacturing Company.
    Bibliography: p.
    Includes index.
    1. Wound healing—Congresses. 2. Wounds—Infections—
Congresses. 3. Wounds—Complications and
sequelae—Congresses. I. Hunt, Thomas K. II. Minne-
sota Mining and Manufacturing Company
RD94.W68   617'.14   79-19835
ISBN 0-8385-9836-6

Text and cover design: Jon Bausch

PRINTED IN THE UNITED STATES OF AMERICA

Contents

Contributors   vii

Preface   xi

1/ Inflammation, Cell Proliferation, and Connective   1
    Tissue Formation in Wound Repair
    Russell Ross

2/ The Physiology of Wound Healing   11
    I. A. Silver

3/ The Biochemical Basis of Repair   32
    D. S. Jackson

4/ Proteoglycans of the Connective Tissue   45
    Ground Substance
    J. Peter Bentley

5/ The Effect of Blood and Oxygen Supply   56
    on the Biochemistry of Repair
    Juha Niinikoski

6/ Atherosclerosis and Healing   72
    C. Heughan, J. Niinikoski, and Thomas K. Hunt

7/ The Healing of Partial-Thickness Skin Injures   81
    Timothy A. Miller

8/ Hormone Influence on Wound Healing   99
    Juhani Ahonen, Hasse Jiborn, and Bengt Zederfeldt

9/ Wound Healing and Diabetes   106
    William H. Goodson, Justin Radolf, and Thomas K.
    Hunt

10/ Collagen Morphology in Normal and Wound Tissue   118
    J. C. Forrester

11/ Zinc and Other Factors of the Pharmacology   135
    of Wound Healing
    M. Chvapil

12/ Colon Repair: The Collagenous Equilibrium   153
    T. K. Hunt, P. R. Hawley, J. Hale, W. Goodson,
    and K. K. Thakral

13/ Problems of Repair in the Colon: Laboratory   **160**
    and Clinical Correlations
    Thomas T. Irvin

14/ Determinants of the Unsuccessful Colonic   **184**
    Anastomosis in Humans
    Theodore R. Schrock

15/ Sutures and Wound Repair   **194**
    James C. Forrester

16/ Skin Closure—Sutures and Tape   **208**
    Juhani Ahonen, Hasse Jiborn, and Bengt Zederfeldt

17/ The Biology of Infections: Sutures, Tapes,   **214**
    and Bacteria
    Richard F. Edlich, George Rodeheaver,
    Gerald T. Golden, and Milton T. Edgerton

18/ Debridement: An Essential Component   **229**
    of Traumatic Wound Care
    Beth Haury, George Rodeheaver, JoAnn Vensko,
    Milton T. Edgerton, and Richard F. Edlich

19/ The Physiology of Wound Infection   **242**
    John F. Burke

20/ Environmental Control of Microbial Contamination   **254**
    in the Operating Room
    Morris L. V. French, Harold E. Eitzen,
    Merrill A. Ritter, and Diane S. Leland

21/ Host Resistance of Infection: Established   **264**
    and Emerging Concepts
    David C. Hohn

22/ Inflammation in Wounds: From "Laudable Pus"   **281**
    to Primary Repair and Beyond
    Thomas K. Hunt and Betty Halliday

Index   **295**

Contributors

Juhani Ahonen, M.D.
Assistant Professor of Surgery, Fourth Department of Surgery, Helsinki University, Helsinki, Finland

J. Peter Bentley, Ph.D.
Professor of Biochemistry, Department of Experimental Biology, University of Oregon Medical School, Portland, Oregon

John F. Burke, M.D.
Professor of Surgery, Harvard Medical School, Massachusetts General Hospital, Boston, Massachusetts

Milos Chvapil, M.D., Ph.D.
Professor of Surgical Biology, Department of Surgery, College of Medicine, Arizona Medical Center, The University of Arizona, Tucson, Arizona

Milton T. Edgerton, M.D.
Professor and Chairman, Department of Plastic Surgery, University of Virginia Medical Center, Charlottesville, Virginia

Richard F. Edlich, M.D., Ph.D.
Assistant Professor of Surgery, Department of Plastic Surgery, University of Virginia Medical Center, Charlottesville, Virginia

Harold E. Eitzen, Ph.D.
Director, Hospital Infection Control, Indiana University School of Medicine, Indianapolis, Indiana

James C. Forrester, M.B., ChM., F.R.C.S.
Senior Lecturer, Department of Surgery, The University of Dundee, Consultant Surgeon, Ninewells Hospital, Dundee, Scotland

Morris L. V. French, Ph.D.
Director of Biology and Serology, Department of Pathology, Indiana University School of Medicine, Indianapolis, Indiana

Gerald T. Golden, M.D.
Instructor in Plastic Surgery, University of Virginia Medical Center, Charlottesville, Virginia

William H. Goodson, III, M.D.
Clinical Instructor in Surgery, Department of Surgery, University of California, San Francisco, California

John E. Hale, M.S., F.R.C.S.
Consultant Surgeon, Department of Surgery, Queen Mary's Hospital, London, England

Betty Halliday, B.A.
Staff Research Associate, Department of Surgery, School of Medicine, University of California, San Francisco, California

Beth Haury, M.A.
Research Assistant, Department of Plastic Surgery, University of Virginia Medical Center, Charlottesville, Virginia

Peter R. Hawley, M.S., F.R.C.S.
Consultant Surgeon, Department of Surgery, St. Mark's Hospital, London, England

Christopher Heughan, F.R.C.S.
Professor of Surgery, Department of Surgery, Memorial University of Newfoundland, St. John's, Newfoundland, Canada

David C. Hohn, M.D.
Assistant Professor of Surgery, Department of Surgery, School of Medicine, University of California, San Francisco, California

Thomas T. Irvin, Ph.D., ChM., F.R.C.S.E.
Senior Lecturer in Surgery, The Royal Infirmary, The University of Sheffield, Sheffield, England

David S. Jackson, Ph.D.
Professor and Chairman, Department of Medical Biochemistry, University of Manchester, Manchester, England

Hasse Jiborn, M.D.
Assistant Professor of Surgery, Department of Surgery, Malmö General Hospital, University of Lund, Malmö, Sweden

Diane S. Leland, M.T., A.S.C.P.
Department of Pathology, Indiana University School of Medicine, Indianapolis, Indiana

Timothy A. Miller, M.D.
Assistant Professor of Surgery, Chief of Plastic Surgery, University of California School of Medicine, Los Angeles, California

Juha Niinikoski, M.D.
Professor of Surgery, Department of Surgery, University of Turku, Turku, Finland

Justin David Radolf, M.D.
Medical Resident in Internal Medicine, Hospital of the University of Pennsylvania, Philadelphia, Pennsylvania.

Merrill A. Ritter, M.D.
Associate Professor, Department of Orthopedic Surgery, Indiana University School of Medicine, Indianapolis, Indiana

George Rodeheaver, Ph.D.
Associate Professor, Department of Plastic Surgery, University of Virginia Medical Center, Charlottesville, Virginia

Russell Ross, Ph.D.
Associate Dean, Scientific Affairs, Department of Pathology, University of Washington School of Medicine, Seattle, Washington

Theodore R. Schrock, M.D.
Associate Professor of Surgery Department of Surgery, University of California, San Francisco, California

Ian A. Silver, M.A., M.R.C.V.S.
Professor of Comparative Pathology, Department of Pathology, University of Bristol, The Medical School, Bristol, England

Kewal K. Thakral, M.D.
Reader in Surgery, State Ayurvedic College, Lucknow, India

JoAnn Vensko, B.S.
Department of Plastic Surgery, University of Virginia Medical Center, Charlottesville, Virginia

Bengt Zederfeldt, M.D.
Professor of Surgery, Department of Surgery, Malmo General Hospital, University of Lund, Malmo, Sweden

Preface

In October 1977 a group of clinicians and investigators interested in wound healing and wound infection met in San Francisco. The symposium was held for two reasons. The first was that it was a good time for active investigators to communicate, and the second was to honor Dr. J.E. Dunphy on the occasion of his retirement from active chairmanship of the Department of Surgery at the University of California, San Francisco.

This book is the outcome of that meeting—a compilation of essays on wounds reflecting not only the recent accomplishments in the field, but the vision and judgment of the participants as well. Although the symposium took place in 1977, the articles in this volume are current. The authors have updated where necesary, and it is a tribute to their foresight that few changes have been necessary.

Many of the contributors owe their start in wound-healing research to Dr. Dunphy's active support in the laboratories of the Boston City Hospital, the University of Oregon, and the University of California. All owe to him an intellectual impetus and a faith that advances in the knowledge of wound healing will inevitably prevent loss of lives and needless suffering. Since he first began his research, he has had the enormous privilege of seeing this faith magnified by accomplishment, and so have we. The goal is now clear—that someday patients (and surgeons) will no longer suffer through failed wounds, leaking anastomoses, and critical wound infections—and we are well along the way.

The editors and participants wish to acknowledge the support of the 3-M Corporation, which sponsored the symposium and made it possible to reassemble many members of "the group" who have scattered to carry their vision through six major countries about the globe. To those who belong to the WWBS (i.e., the "Worked With Bert" Society), but could not participate, we send our grief at their loss of a fine week in San Francisco, our sorrow at not having their fellowship there, our joy in recalling the hours we spent together in the laboratories, and our admonition to keep plugging.

In recent years, Dr. Dunphy has done no active "bench" research, but during that time, he gave us something which is equally important. As Kahlil Gibran wrote in *the Prophet:*

> No man can reveal to you aught but that which already lies half asleep in the dawning of your knowledge.
>
> The teacher who walks in the shadow of the temple, among his followers, gives not of his wisdom, but rather of his faith and his lovingness.
>
> If he is indeed wise he does not bid you enter the house of his wisdom, but rather leads you to the threshold of your own mind. . . .
>
> And even as each one of you stands alone in God's knowledge, so must each one of you be alone in his knowledge of God and in his understanding of the earth.

Thomas K. Hunt
San Francisco, 1979

Wound Healing and Wound Infection

Inflammation, Cell Proliferation, and Connective Tissue Formation in Wound Repair

1

Russell Ross

The process of wound repair, whether the healing be of primary or secondary intention, has long been known to consist of a chronological sequence of events characterized by the various cellular infiltrates that appear within the wound. This sequence was recognized many years ago by Metchnikoff[1] and was quantified in primary wound repair by Ross and Benditt.[2] This review will attempt to place in perspective those cellular events that are recognized to be important, clarify what is known about the interrelationships between the various cell types that appear during the process of inflammation and wound repair, and indicate the directions that new research will undoubtedly take.

THE SEQUENCE OF WOUND REPAIR

Immediately after wounding, the process of coagulation involves both the humoral aspects of coagulation and the cellular response. The principal cellular response concerns the interaction of the platelets with thrombin and collagen. These small cells have long been recognized to play a primary role in coagulation, both by mechanically adhering to one another to induce cessation of hemorrhage and by providing components and initiators of the intrinsic process of coagulation. Recently, it has been recognized that these cells contain substances that may play an important role in wound repair.

Once the coagulation process is completed, the various types of leukocytes appear in the wound in an orderly and reproducible sequence.[2,3] The earliest cells to appear are the polymorphonuclear neutrophils (granulocytes) and the blood monocytes. On entering the wound, the latter become the principal macrophages responsible for debriding the wound.[1,3,4] Neutrophils appear within a few hours, remain in large numbers for another day or two, and then rapidly decline in number if there is no concomitant infection. Monocytes enter the wounds and rapidly modulate into macrophages, reaching their maximal number some 24 hours later than do the neutrophils and decreasing in number slightly later. A significant number of macrophages persist even in primarily closed wounds for at least several weeks and longer in open or dead-space wounds.

Fibroblasts and capillaries appear in the wound slightly later than leukocytes. In linear incisions, the fibroblasts begin to appear within one day and become maximal in number within one week to 10 days; capillaries follow in a similar time course. The fibroblasts are responsible for the formation of the connective tissue components, specifically, collagen and the glycosaminoglycans (mucopolysaccharides), and, at a much later stage, for the formation of elastic fibers. Initially, it was thought that elastic fibers do not form in the process of wound repair, but Williams[5] has recently shown that new elastic fibers can be found in scars that are 60 days or older. Consequently, elastic fiber formation must be considered a part of the process of wound repair and scar formation.

During the process of resolution and remodeling to form the final scar, the highly cellular granulation tissue becomes transformed into a relatively acellular mass, and a majority of the fibroblasts and capillaries disappear. One of the significant unresolved questions concerning the process of wound remodeling and the relative acellular appearance of the final scar relates to the mode of the disappearance of fibroblasts and capillaries.

The hallmark of granluation tissue is the marked proliferative response of the fibroblasts that is accompanied by the formation of new capillaries and by the synthesis and secretion of large amounts of connective tissue matrix components.

A number of important questions have been raised concerning the significance of the sequence of the appearance of the cells during the process of wound repair: Is this sequence obligatory? Must neutrophils appear before monocytes? Must monocytes appear before fibroblasts? Do some of these cells participate in the appearance of the others? Is this a single sequence or do each of the cells have an independent function?

THROMBOCYTE

Although the blood platelet has long been recognized to be important in the process of coagulation, it has recently been noted that the many granules present in the platelets are rich in lysosomal enzymes, adenosine triphosphate (ATP), serotonin, and "growth factors." The presence of growth factors in platelets has only been recognized within the past two years. They were discovered in a series of studies of the control of proliferation of smooth muscle cells and fibroblasts in cell culture.[6-9]

All diploid cells in culture require some form of serum to be present in the culture medium for the cells to synthesize DNA and increase in number. Many attempts have been made to characterize the factors,[10,11,12] but their source had not been well explained. Some of them are insulinlike in their characteristics, whereas others act more like a growth hormone.

In 1973, Ross et al.[6] and Rutherford and Ross[7] discovered that when smooth muscle cells or fibroblasts were grown in culture in the presence of cell-free, plasma-derived serum, rather than whole-blood serum, the cells would remain quiescent in culture for extended periods of time. Furthermore, they were able to demonstrate that the addition of platelets purified from the pool of blood from which the cell-free plasma-derived serum was made could restore all of the proliferative capacity present in the whole blood serum that was missing in the plasma-derived serum. To further prove that the mitogenic capacity of whole blood serum was the result of a factor released from thrombocytes, Ross et al.[6] exposed a purified preparation of thrombocytes to purified bovine thrombin in a separate series of in vitro experiments. Platelets that had released their components after exposure to thrombin were removed, and the supernatant from the release reaction was added to previously formed cell-free, plasma-derived serum. This supernatant, which restored all of the mitogenic capacity of whole-blood serum to fibroblasts and smooth muscle cells in culture, is derived from the physiological response of platelet aggregation and release that results from platelet exposure to collagen or thrombin. Work is going forward to further characterize the platelet mitogenic factor(s).

All blood serum, by definition, must contain platelet-derived factors. Since plasma serum lacks the proliferative capacity of blood serum, the principal mitogenic characteristics of whole blood serum must be platelet-derived.

It has also been recently shown that platelets act in vivo to provide mitogenic factors to stimulate smooth muscle cells to proliferate.[8] Studies are underway to determine whether the platelet factors play a similar role in healing wounds. These studies should further our understanding of the nature of the initiating factors that stimulate the first round of fibroblast proliferation and wound repair. They would suggest that perhaps a principal, early initiating factor is thrombocyte derived.

THE NEUTROPHIL

The early appearance of the polymorphonuclear neutrophilic leukocyte during wound repair, which is followed in an orderly manner by monocytes and fibroblasts, suggests that this sequence may also be obligatory. In a series of studies, Simpson and Ross[9] were able to induce a selective neutropenia in guinea pigs by daily administration of an antineutrophil serum. This serum was highly specific for neutrophils, so much so that it did not cross-react with eosinophils or basophils. In animals kept in a relative pathogen-free state, it was possible to induce a neutropenia for a period of 10 days by daily administration of antineutrophil serum. Thus, they were able to examine the process of wound repair in the absence of any circulating neutrophils. No neutrophils were present in any of the wounds throughout the 10-day period. There was no alteration in the sequence of the appearance of monocytes, fibroblasts, and capillaries or in the formation of collagen. These studies demonstrated that the neutrophil is not a necessary antecedent in wound repair in the absence of overt infection. If relatively small numbers of microorganisms were present in the wounds, the macrophages appeared to be capable of handling them. In the presence of large numbers of bacteria, the wounds went on to become infected and the animals died of septicemia and bacteremia.

The results presented here are in contrast to earlier studies[13] that suggested that the neutrophil was a necessary antecedent in the chronology of the appearance of the cells. They are supported by the observations of Hill and Ward[14] and Dale and Wolff[15] in which the healing process following myocardial infarction or implanted skin windows was studied. In both instances, selective neutropenia had no effect on the process of fibrosis.

Consequently, the neutrophil is clearly an important first line of defense in the presence of infection. It appears, however, to play no role in stimulating the appearance of the cells that enter the wound at later time intervals.

COMPLEMENT

In a similarly designed series of studies, Wahl et al.[16] examined the process of wound repair in animals that had been decomplemented by the use of cobra venom factor. The observations in their studies were essentially unaltered. The animals did show a decrease in the number of neutrophils in the wounds, but, as in the earlier studies in the neutropenic animals, this had no effect upon the process of wound repair. Consequently, complement does not appear to play a major role in the healing process in the absence of overt infection.

THE MONONUCLEAR PHAGOCYTE

The observations eliminating both the neutrophil and complement as critical elements in the chronology of wound repair suggested that the blood monocyte might be important in the healing process.

The source of the wound fibroblast has long been a controversial topic. Much of the early literature stated that the fibroblast was derived from the blood monocyte. In an early sequence of studies, Volkman and Gowans[17,18] demonstrated in parabiotic rats that macrophages present in inflammatory responses, including the healing wound, are derived from blood-borne monocytes. Ross et al.[19] used a similar technique in Lewis strain inbred rats to determine whether wound fibroblasts were derived from the monocyte. In the parabiotic rat, it is possible to label the blood monocytes from one donor animal and to follow these labeled monocytes as they appear in wounds in an irradiated parabiotic mate. In such a situation, none of the white blood cells in the wound can be derived from the marrow of the irradiated parabiont but must come from its unirradiated mate. By labeling the cells from the nonirradiated donor with tritiated thymidine, it was possible to follow their presence by both light and electron microscope autoradiography in the irradiated recipient. These studies demonstrated that isotopically labeled neutrophils, lymphocytes, and monocytes were able to cross the circulation into the unlabeled irradiated parabiont and were found in its wound. At no time were labeled fibroblasts present in the wounds of the irradiated parabiont—although its wounds contained large numbers of fibroblasts—and the process of wound repair was unaltered. These studies demonstrated that the fibroblasts were not derived from circulating monocytes and suggested that they came from cells in the adjacent intact connective tissues surrounding the wound.

When it was demonstrated that wound fibroblasts were not derived from blood monocytes, another series of studies was pursued to determine whether the blood monocyte provided components in the wound that stimulated the process of fibroblast migration and proliferation. To perform these studies, Leibovich and Ross[20] used several means of interfering with macrophage function to determine the importance of these cells.

An antimacrophage serum was developed which in cell culture was capable of paralyzing monocytes or macrophages so that they were no longer capable of phagocytosis. Leibovich and Ross[3] took advantage of the earlier observations by Van Furth and his colleagues,[21] who observed that the administration of hydrocortisone would induce a monocytopenia. They made guinea pigs monocytopenic in this manner and proceeded to study wound repair in four groups of animals. These included

1. Control animals
2. Animals made monocytopenic with hydrocortisone
3. Animals containing antimacrophage serum injections subcutaneously around the wound
4. Animals made monocytopenic with hydrocortisone and injected with antimacrophage serum subcutaneously around the wound

Each animal contained six linear incisions in its dorsal skin. The wounds were examined after various time intervals, and the number of cells was quantified at each point in time by both light and electron microscopy. In these studies, Leibovich and Ross[3] observed that the only group that showed a modulation of the process of wound repair were those that were made monocytopenic and whose macrophages were paralyzed by periwound subcutaneous administration of antimacrophage serum. In these circumstances, the processes of fibroblast migration and proliferation and connective tissue formation were markedly delayed, suggesting that the macrophage indeed played an important role that precedes the appearance of fibroblasts and connective tissue formation in the wounds.

These studies led to a series of cell-culture experiments in which Leibovich and Ross[20] demonstrated that when stimulated macrophages secrete a component that will initiate DNA synthesis and cell division when exposed to wound fibroblasts in culture. These experiments took advantage of the fact that fibroblasts will not proliferate in a culture medium containing platelet-poor, plasma-derived serum. They incubated macrophages in a similar medium and then exposed these macrophages to latex particles or to other factors that would stimulate the macrophages to become phagocytic. Six hours after stimulation, the medium was removed from the macrophages and was fed to fibroblasts that had been quiescent in similar medium. Shortly after, the cells were exposed to the medium that had seen the activated macrophages. The fibroblasts were stimulated into logarithmic growth and extensive proliferation. These studies suggested that the macrophage activation somehow led to the production of a component in the culture medium that stimulated fibroblast growth. Work is underway to determine the nature of the component formed by the macrophages and its mode of action on other cells.

FURTHER DIRECTIONS

Future research should clarify the role of platelets in the initiation of cell proliferation in wound repair and should determine the various roles played by macrophages beyond that of phagocytosis and wound debridement. The experiments suggesting that macrophages are important in stimulating fibroplasia could be of fundamental importance because of the ubiquitious role of these cells in many tissue alterations. The isolation, characterization, and identification of the macrophage factor(s) will be critical in understanding these events.

Little is known concerning the factors that control collagen synthesis. Collagen is the principal connective tissue component of the healing wound, and it will be necessary to further pursue the nature of the factors responsible for stimulating collagen formation by, and proliferation of, fibroblasts. These and other studies could provide a basis for the manipulation of the process of wound repair in terms of rapidity, the extent of scar formation, and the prevention of faulty healing.

REFERENCES

1. Metchnikoff E: Lectures on the Comparative Pathology of Inflammation. Starling FA, Starling EH, trans. New York, Dover, 1891
2. Ross R, Benditt EP: Wound healing and collagen formation I. Sequential changes in components of guinea pig skin wounds observed in the electron microscope. J Biophys Biochem Cytol 11:677, 1961
3. Leibovich SJ, Ross R: The role of the macrophage in wound repair: Study with hydrocortisone and anti-macrophage serum. Am J Pathol 78:71, 1975
4. Ross R: The fibroblast and wound repair. Biol Rev 43:51, 1968
5. Williams G: The late phases of wound healing: Histological and ultrastructural studies of collagen and elastic-tissue formation. J Pathol 102:61, 1970
6. Ross R, Glomset J, Kariya B, Harker L: A platelet-dependent serum factor

that stimulates the proliferation of arterial smooth muscle cells *in vitro*. Proc Natl Acad Sci USA 71:1207, 1974

7. Rutherford R, Ross R: Platelet factors stimulate fibroblasts and smooth muscle cells quiescent in plasma-serum to proliferate. J Cell Biol 69:196, 1976

8. Harker L, Ross R, Slichter S, Scott C: Homocystine-induced arteriosclerosis: The role of endothelial cell injury and platelet response in its genesis. J Clin Invest 58:731, 1976

9. Simpson D, Ross R: The neutrophilic leukocyte in wound repair: A study with anti-neutrophil serum. J Clin Invest 51:2009, 1972

10. Castor LN: Control of division by cell contact and serum concentration in cultures of 373 cells. Exp Cell Res 68:17, 1971

11. Kohler N, Lipton A: Platelets as a source of fibroblast growth promoting activity. Exp Cell Res 87:297, 1974

12. Westermark B, Wasteson A: A platelet factor stimulating human glial cells. Exp Cell Res 98:170, 1976

13. Page AR, Good RA: A clinical and experimental study of the function of neutrophils in the inflammatory response. Am J Pathol 34:645, 1968

14. Hill JH, Ward PA: The phlogistic role of leukotactic fragments in myocardial infarcts of rats. J Exp Med 133:885, 1971

15. Dale DC, Wolff SM: Skin window studies of the acute inflammatory responses of neutropenic patients. Blood 38:138, 1971

16. Wahl S, Arend WP, Ross R: The effect of complement depletion on wound healing. Am J Pathol 74:73, 1974

17. Volkman A, Gowans JL: The production of macrophages in the rat. Br J Exp Pathol 46:50, 1965

18. Volkman A, Gowans JL: The origin of macrophages from bone marrow in the rat. Br J Exp Pathol 46:62, 1965

19. Ross R, Everett NB, Tyler R: Wound healing and collagen formation. VI. The origin of the wound fibroblast studied in parabiosis. J Cell Biol 44:645, 1970

20. Leibovich SJ, Ross R: A macrophage dependent factor that stimulates the proliferation of fibroblasts *in vitro*. Am J Pathol 84:501, 1976

21. Thomas J, Van Furth R: The effect of glucocorticosteroids on the kinetics of mononuclear phagocytes. J Exp Med 131:429, 1970

Comment

In this remarkably brief and clear essay, Dr. Ross has sketched in the current knowledge about the details of what used to be known as the "lag phase" of wound healing. The older name obtained its dignity through the observation that wounds gained little tensile strength in the first few days after closure. The name stuck, despite the fact that many investigators pointed out that the "lag phase" was actually one of intense activity. Sandburg and associates showed that delaying the inflammatory response with steroids delays repair. However, if steroids are not given until the inflammatory phase has occurred, wound healing is disturbed very little. We can conclude from this that there is something essential about inflammation and that wound healing is a sequence in which injury is the first step, inflammation the second, and fibroplasia the third. The evaluation of this idea parallels the development of surgery and is presented in more detail in Chapter 22.

Several investigators, notably Stein and Levenson (1976), have shown that granulocytes and lymphocytes play little role in uncomplicated repair; others, particularly Fromer and Klintworth (1976) felt that granulocytes excite angiogenesis in the cornea. Our experiences (see Chapter 22) tend to agree with those of Dr. Ross. The macrophage seems to be a mysterious and plenipotential cell!

These studies have initiated a new era in the investigation of repair. For the first time we are learning what aspects of injury lead to scar formation. If you reflect for a moment, you will remember that mechanical, thermal, or chemical injury are not the only ways to activate a macrophage or deposit a platelet in a small vessel. Obviously, an immune reaction can activate a macrophage, and in these studies we see a point at which immune and granulomatous inflammation and wound healing merge in a final common pathway which expresses the natural result of these primary events, i.e., scar formation. Dr. Ross has also shown elsewhere that defective endothelium can attract platelets which can then elicit a fibroblastic response. After many years in which all wound-healing investigation concentrated on collagen as the important substance in repair, these studies have finally turned to cells as the "intelligent agents." In these simple, elegant experiments Dr. Ross has outlined a sequence from injury to blood clot to inflammation to fibrogenesis. This sequence will be discussed further in later chapters.

In his closing remarks, Dr. Ross writes of stimulators of collagen synthesis. He points out that it is one thing to cause a fibroblast to multiply and migrate toward an injury, but it may be quite another to cause it to synthesize and deposit collagen. Evidence is already accumulating that other signals are involved, and this, too, will be covered in a later chapter. In view of a later essay by Heughan on some similarities between arteriosclerosis and wound healing, it seems appropriate to add two of Dr. Ross's classic papers to the reference list (Ross and Glomset 1976a,b).

ADDITIONAL REFERENCES

Fromer C, Klintworth GK: Studies related to the vasoproliferative capability of leukocytes and leukocyte components. Am J Pathol 82:157, 1976

Ross R, Glomset JA: The pathogenesis of atherosclerosis. Part 1. N Engl J Med 295:369, 1976a

Ross R, Glomset JA: The pathogenesis of atherosclerosis. Part 2. N Engl J Med 295:420, 1976b

Stein JM, Levenson SM: Effect of the inflammatory resection on subsequent healing. Surg Forum 17:484, 1966

The Physiology of Wound Healing
2

I. A. Silver

The repair of damage is a fundamental quality of living tissue, but its method of expression is a compromise between the competing needs of different cell types, e.g., those of epidermis versus connective tissue or of hard tissue versus soft tissue. The study of the environmental conditions under which cell and tissue repair take place is relatively recent and has been pioneered especially by Hunt and his group in San Francisco (Hunt and Hutchison 1966; Hunt et al. 1967, 1968, 1969; Hunt and Zederfeldt 1969) and by Niinikoski and associates in Turku, Finland (Kulonen and Niinikoski 1968; Niinikoski and Kulonen 1970; Niinikoski 1969). The development of micro techniques for the direct measurement of physical environment at the cellular level has enabled much more precise determination of the conditions under which the cells live, both in culture and in tissues (Remensnyder and Majno 1968; Silver 1965, 1966, 1969, 1973a, 1973b, 1975). This chapter outlines the cellular events that take place during wound healing and how these events may be altered by the presence of infection or foreign bodies and by vascular disturbances such as hemorrhagic shock. Consideration is given only to the healing of skin wounds with the main emphasis on the connective tissue component.

GENERAL DISCUSSION

Cellular Events

When skin is damaged the following events take place:
 Hemorrhage leads to the formation of a clot with a fibrin framework

11

which dries and contracts and which may act to some extent as a glue to hold the clot to the surface of the tissue. In open wounds it fails to protect underlying tissue from the dehydration resulting from evaporation of water vapor through the clot in the initial phase of scab formation. The clot and scab give immediate, if relatively poor, mechanical protection against ingress of foreign material such as dust or bacteria to the wound surface (see Comment).

An inflammatory response develops, the extent and severety of which depends on the type of wound. In burns the cellular phase of the inflammatory reaction may be delayed or even almost absent.

After a period of 4 to 6 hours, epithelial cells at the edges of the wound can be seen to accumulate glycogen granules, and after a further 4 to 6 hours mitoses appear in the basal layers of the epithelium and cells begin to migrate from these layers, either under the edges of the clot or across or through it, depending on how much dehydration has taken place. The migration of the epithelium is by a "leap-frogging" process in which the mobile cells do not lose contact with the previous fixed epithelial cells. A basement membrane reaction forms between epithelium and connective tissue immediately after a cell has settled in to its new position. During the migration process, epithelial cells may cut through the collagen of the dermis, presumably by means of collagenases either secreted by themselves or activated in the tissues through which they are passing. It is worthy of note that epithelial cells will migrate through intact established dermis but will not pass through healthy granulation tissue. When they meet granulation tissue, they become deflected over its surface (see Chapter 7).

During the early phase after wounding, and continuing until closure, there is a progressive contraction of fibroblasts in the area deep to the wound leading to primary wound contraction under the influence of inflammatory secretions on their myofibrils (Gabbiani et al. 1973).

After a period of between 24 and 36 hours, the first signs of proliferative connective tissue activity can be seen; these consist of division of the fibroblasts and endothelial cells. Prior to this proliferation, cells have been accumulating in the connective tissue through the inflammatory reaction which occurs around a wound, and by 24 to 36 hours the early predominance of the polymorphonuclear cell has been overtaken by the accumulation of macrophages. The macrophages move into the area of damaged tissue and into the clot, which they remove by phagocytosis (see Comment). The new connective tissue cells follow the macrophages and migrate into the space that has been cleared. The usual arrangement in regenerating connective tissue is that the macrophages form an "advance guard" which is followed shortly by endothelial buds which grow in arcades to join each other and then become canalized. These endothelial arcades are clothed by mesenchyme cells which are visually undifferentiated but which can be shown by immunofluorescent anticollagen antibody staining to produce a protocollagen. They must therefore be classified as some kind of fibroblast. These three cell types—the macrophage, the endothelial cell, and the fibroblast—make up the majority of granulation tissue which has the key role in the healing of all organs except those of epithelial origin. Granulation tissue is highly vascular, delicate, and easily damaged; it is extremely resistant to infection; and it will ultimately change to scar tissue. In wounds where irritation persists the granulation tissue may also contain significant numbers of constantly replaced polymorphs, and, if there is immunological aspect to the irritation, plasma cells, lymphocytes, and eosinophil leukocytes may also be present in large numbers. Granulation tissue grows to fill all the spaces available to it but does not usually grow beyond the normal level of the epithelial line. We are still without an explanation as to why connective tissue growth ceases at this particular point, but it is clearly associated with the presence of a complete epithelial covering. As the granulation tissue fills the wound cavity, the older parts of it become organized in such a way that the fibroblasts that are left behind synthesize more collagen around themselves and fibrillar collagen polymerizes from the extracellular protocollagen. These fibrils then cross-link to a greater or lesser extent depending on the situation (see Chapter 3). As time passes, more and more collagen and proteoglycans are laid down in relation to the number of cells present; finally, the blood supply tends to close down, although "ghosts" of small vessels are present among the mature fibers. It should perhaps be emphasized that the blood clot does not form a scaffolding on which repair takes place. The presence of a solid clot is an inhibitory factor in healing and delays the formation of granulation tissue, but small amounts of blood containing platelets, together with the macrophages, appear to be stimulatory (Ordman and Gillman 1966a, b, c) (see Comment).

The Stimulus to Repair

A large number of theories have been produced to account for the repair of tissue. These may be listed as follows:

A positive stimulus may result from the release of some factor by the wounding of tissue. These factors have been called wound hormones or trephones (Abercrombie 1957; Hell 1970). This view has received a renewed impetus following recent observations on the possible functions of blood platelets in wounds (see Chapter 1).

The removal of an inhibitory feedback mechanism has been thought to allow healing. This has been described particularly by Bullough and

Lawrence (1966) who have identified mitotic inhibitory substances in mature cells which they have called *chalones*, from the Greek word meaning "bridle." In this view, as they age and as part of their normal metabolism, cells produce a mitotic inhibitory substance which not only prevents the aging cell itself from dividing but may diffuse out from the cell when it dies or loses membrane integrity, thus reducing the mitotic activity of cells around it. The most convincing evidence for the presence of chalone has been found in the epidermis, where it has been shown that a substance can be extracted from the superficial layers of the epidermis which inhibits the activity of the basal cells. This material is similar whether it comes from a codfish, a mouse, or a human, but it has no effect on cells other than those of squamous epithelium. Other chalones affecting connective tissue cells have also been found (Bullough 1965, 1971; Bullough and Lawrence 1968, 1970; Cross 1972; Marks 1972).

Physical factors have been suggested as being involved in stimulating repair. Among these have been altered gradients of oxygen tension, pH or ionic concentrations, particularly potassium released from damaged cells (Silver 1975; Maroudas 1975), and mechanical effects, such as changes of tension, which may occur in damaged tissue.

Biological factors have been proposed, e.g., cell hypoxia resulting from damaged blood supply. This has been a popular suggestion since it can be seen that new blood vessels tend to grow towards hypoxic areas. Recent evidence, however, has suggested that the macrophage may be a very important part of the stimulus to repair and may indeed produce gradients in some way. Possibly, macrophages emerging into damaged tissue through the inflammatory reaction become "activated" during their removal of debris and release some substance which diffuses back into the normal tissue, thereby creating a chemotaxic gradient and stimulating the migration of fibroblasts and endothelial cells towards the damaged area, and possibly their division. (Clark et al. 1976). It might also be suggested that a macrophage which has been in contact with tissue debris may become "primed" by such contact and pass on a message to endothelial cells and fibroblasts through direct contact by a mechanism similar to that whereby macrophages are known to process antigens and pass on information about their structure to lymphocytes prior to antibody production in lymph nodes.

We have the problem of the burn as a peculiar wound that does not heal easily. So far, there is no clear and generally accepted explanation of the slow healing of burns, but it seems quite likely that either the lack of a clear edge to the injury fails to stimulate the necessary inflammation and repair response or, alternatively, there is an inhibition of these responses by some toxic by-products that diffuse out of the burn tissue. In addition, heat-coagulated tissue, and especially collagen, appears to be difficult for macrophages to remove.

Scar Formation

The end result of the connective tissue healing process is the formation of scar tissue from granulation tissue. Collagen arrangement in a scar is different from that in normal tissue but, nevertheless, the collagen present in the scar is turned over by fibroblasts at much the same rate as the normal (see Chapter 3). During this turnover there is long-term change in cross-linking of fiber arrangement and there can be a reorganization of the fiber direction of the scar, particularly in places where there are mechanical stresses placed on the wound. A feature of epithelium over scars is that the thickness is usually rather less than normal and the attachment to the underlying scar is less effective than it is in normal tissue because the rete pegs are short and sparse. Therefore, the epithelium is relatively easily eroded by friction, and furthermore, because of the poor blood supply of scar tissue, and thus to its epithelium, pressure necrosis is very easily produced.

Having touched briefly on some aspects of general interest in wound healing, we turn to a more detailed consideration of experimental findings in wounds.

CELLULAR MICROENVIRONMENT IN WOUND HEALING

For a rational approach to the treatment of any kind of wound, it is necessary to know what cellular events are taking place within the wound at different stages in the healing process. It is difficult to get a continous assessment of this process through histological sections since these give only a series of "stills" in an ongoing process and, therefore, a nondestructive model is needed. We have used an almost two-dimensional model in the form of a wound in the transparent rabbit ear chamber. This technique allows measurement of the physical environment and also continuous photographic records and direct microscopic observation of the various cells and fibers that are formed during healing.

METHODS

Plastic chambers, derived from an orginal design of Sumner and Wood (Wood et al. 1966) but made of polymethylpentene (TPX) or polycarbonate—which are biologically compatible, almost completely trans-

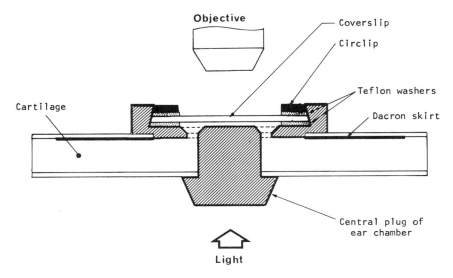

FIG. 1. *Cross-sectional diagram of ear chamber, in relation to microscopic examination. New tissue grows into the space between the "plug" and the coverslip, the depth of which is determined by the thickness of the Teflon spacer.*

parent materials—were turned in a single piece from 20-mm rod and were inserted into the ears of half-lop rabbits. The depth of the cavity within the chamber was determined by the thickness of the "spacer" ring, as can be seen in Figure 1. Two standard spacers were used, one of 12μ and the other of 100μ. The first allowed only capillary networks and very small arterioles and venules to grow onto the table, while the second permitted the development of larger vessels. Invasion by granulation tissue onto the table took place through the holes in the edge of the chamber. It was difficult to induce epithelium to grow in these chambers unless access of air was permitted, in which case vessel development ceased and connective tissue growth usually stopped. We therefore confined our observations with this system to the physiology of the environment in regenerating connective tissue.

By manipulation of the cover slips on the top of the chamber, so that the two holes (Fig. 2) coincided, it was possible to insert probes into the tissue and to make measurements under direct microscopic observation with which every part of the healing system was being examined (Silver 1969). For instance, oxygen environment in the wound space, at the growing edge of the tissue, in the differentiating zone, and in the fully formed fibrous tissue could all be observed through the same hole. Electrodes sensitive to pH, pK, PCO_2, or glucose could also be inserted into the tissue by the same route for making intracellular or extracellular measurements (Silver 1973b, 1976; Thomas 1970, 1976; Zeuthen et al. 1974). Fluorescent-labeled anticollagen antibodies could be introduced to the chamber either systemically through the arterial supply or by removing the cover slip and flooding the area directly with the antibody. The position of adherence of the antibody to the antigen was seen by examining both the chamber under incident ultraviolet light and identified sites of early collagen formation.

Changes in local environment were imposed on the cells in the chamber either by direct application of different gas mixtures to the tissue surface when the coverslip was removed or by altering the systemic situation by varying the gases supplied for respiration. Local blood flow was measured by hydrogen clearance with microgenerating and -detecting platinum electrodes (Lübbers and Baumgärtl 1967; Baumgärtl and Lübbers 1973) and could be altered by compressing the blood supply, so that either arterial ischemia or venous congestion was developed. The effects of hemorrhagic or septic shock or the development of local infection were studied in regard to their ability to alter physiological conditions in the wound and the rate of wound healing. The system was also useful for looking at burns, since the local heating of tissue that had grown within the chamber could be adjusted to produce all stages of thermal damage.

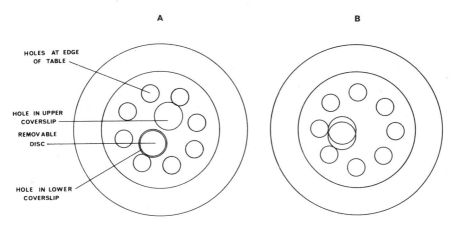

FIG 2. *Surface views of chamber with two coverslips showing how eccentric holes in the coverslips may allow access to the majority of the tissue in the chamber for insertion of electrodes of fluorescent probes.*

RESULTS

The Wound Cavity

Measurements in the wound cavity indicated that there was an early fall in oxygen tension and a rise in PCO_2 together with an increased hydrogen- and potassium-ion concentration during the first few hours after wounding. The PO_2 fell to a minimum of between 10 mm Hg and zero; the exact level seemed to depend on the degree of cellular response to injury and the amount of damage to the blood vessels at the edge of the wound. PO_2 remained low in the cavity until granulation tissue had almost filled the wound space.

PCO_2 rose during the first day or two after wounding and then remained relatively constant at 55 to 65 mm Hg. It began to fall when an

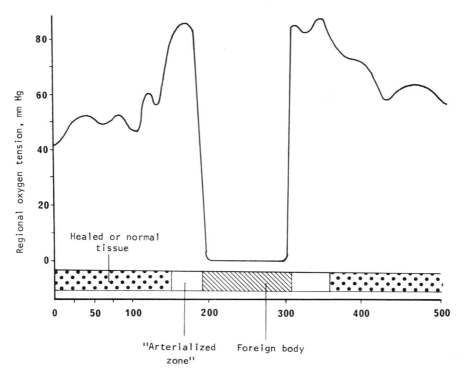

FIG 3.   *Oxygen tension profile across tissue containing a foreign body (horizontal scale in microns). Note the low oxygen content of the foreign body in spite of the increased vascularization in its vicinity.*

active circulation in the new capillaries had been developed and when most of the debris had been removed from the wound cavity. The level of pH was more varied and seemed to depend particularly on the constancy of perfusion of the capillaries at the edge of the wound and the numbers of macrophages in the dead space. Dramatic falls in pH occurred during local ischemia or generalized hypovolemia. The development of the inflammatory response was accompanied by rapid changes of PO_2 which ultimately resulted in a generalized lowering of the oxygen tension in the inflamed tissue. In contaminated wounds bacterial growth produced major changes in environment partly on account of the bacterial activity itself and partly because of the activity of macrophages and other phagocytic cells. Foreign bodies within tissue or in a wound cavity were rapidly surrounded by macrophages and eventually by giant cells. The effect of the cellular activity was to withdraw oxygen from the foreign body and to prevent access of oxygen into it. This cellular response led to ideal conditions for the development of anaerobic bacteria within foreign bodies (Fig. 3).

The Growing Edge of the Wound

At the edge of the proliferating tissue, sprouting capillary buds are found, which are clothed in a layer of cells which appear to be young fibroblasts and macrophages. The macrophage vanguard removed debris and allowed the endothelial shoots to push into a preformed fluid-filled space. Endothelial buds and fibroblasts did not invade solid material such as a blood clot if it was left in a wound. Debris was removed or liquified by macrophages before new tissue was formed. Macrophage activity, as regards removal of debris, occurred efficiently under either aerobic or anaerobic conditions and proceeded equally satisfactorily over a wide range of pH and PO_2. If bacteria were present, however, macrophages were less effective in their role as destroyers of organisms in hypoxic as compared with well-oxygenated situations. Oxygen is presumably necessary for the full deployment of the peroxidases, which constitute one of the mechanisms used in destroying phagocytosed organisms (see Chapters 21 and 22). In hypoxic wounds, macrophages could sometimes be seen to engulf bacterial particles, to carry them in their cytoplasm, and to eject them undamaged. However, if the cells were subsequently provided with oxygen the bacteria still within phagosomes very soon became lysed and disappeared.

Immediately behind the macrophage "screen" were groups of cells which were rounded or slightly elongated and which appeared to have little intercellular matrix. Most of these cells did not show mitoses

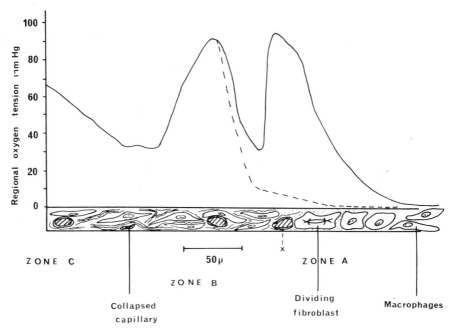

FIG 4.   *Diagrammatic section through new tissue growing in an ear chamber, with oxygen tension profile superimposed. Mitotic activity is almost confined to the leading capillary zone. Collagen cross-linking is occurring in the zone of shallow oxygen gradients. Zone A is the growth zone. Zone B is the "synthetic" zone. Zone C is the established zone. In shock or hypovolemia, if capillary "X" is underperfused the O₂ profile changes to that shown by dashed line.*

unless they were situated close to capillary loops containing circulating blood (Fig. 4). However, if FITC-labelled antisoluble collagen was introduced into this region and the cells were then examined under UV fluorescence, it became clear that they did, in fact, possess a thin surrounding layer of some form of collagen which was antigenically recognizable (Fig. 5). One must assume, therefore, that these were fibroblasts or primitive mesenchyme cells. Growth in the repairing tissue was confined to division of endothelial cells and of fibroblasts associated with them. The region of dividing fibroblastic cells seemed to be limited to a zone of oxygen tension which was of the order of 30–80 mm Hg. Almost no division figures could be found where the oxygen tension was consistently below 25 mm. The CO_2 levels in the dividing zone were intermediate between those in the wound dead space and those in the capillary blood supply.

   A point which may be of some importance clinically is that both hypovolemia and, conversely, the overloading of the circulation with small excesses of saline led to dramatic changes in the environmental conditions of the proliferating zone in wounds. The new capillaries were extremely sensitive to conditions which altered tissue perfusion.

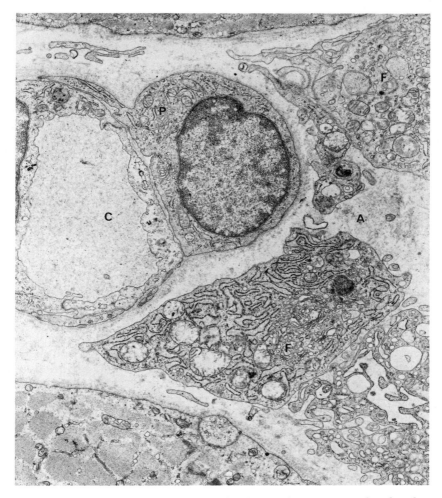

FIG 5.   *Low-power electron micrograph of granulation tissue that has been subjected to 3 hours of hemorrhagic shock. A, antigenically recognizable procollagen; F, young fibroblasts (note mitochondrial damage due to shock); C, capillary; P, pericyte (note that mitochondria in this cell are intact).*

In hypovolemia the capillary loops closed and the growing area became nonperfused. If, on the other hand, the circulation was overloaded, even to a very small extent, with fluid of low colloid osmotic pressure to combat hypovolemia, microedema developed in the growing area when the circulation was restored. This increased the diffusion distances between the capillaries and the growing tissue which, in turn, resulted in hypoxia among the cells not immediately adjacent to capillaries and a subsequent reduction in their mitotic rate.

The Synthetic Zone

Further from the wound edge, towards the normal tissue, the capillaries were less "leaky" and were of normal structure, while the fibroblasts left behind in this region assumed an elongated shape and were surrounded by obvious collagen fibrils. These fibrils became denser toward the periphery of the wound and formed the basis of the repair tissue, which would later undergo contraction. The maximum synthetic and collagen cross-linking activity appeared to take place in a zone in which the oxygen tension was 15–30 mm Hg and where the oxygen diffusion gradients were much less steep than those at the wound edge (see Fig. 4).

Effects of Shock

Hemorrhage of a quite minor nature resulted in the withdrawal of circulation from the growing edge of healing tissue. This occurred well before there was any drop in blood pressure and certainly well before clinical shock was established. Reinfusion of the animal with blood at this stage led to an almost immediate restoration of the circulation through the wound tissue. If hypovolemia was allowed to continue for a longer period until the point at which clinical shock developed, restoration of the blood volume was not then followed by the reopening of the new capillary circulation in the wound edge. In the rabbit, which is rather susceptible to hemorrhage, brief periods of reversible shock could lead to a condition in which new tissue remained underperfused for several days after the restoration of blood volume. This resulted in considerable slowing of the healing process. Since fibroblastic and endothelial proliferation do not normally take place on any large scale until about the third day after wounding, shock occurring at the moment the animal was traumatized and then corrected did not delay healing; if hypovolemia was not recognized, however, or was allowed to persist or develop after the first two days following wounding, this was invariably followed by a considerable delay in the healing process. The effect of shock on the microenvironment was to reduce the oxygen tension to zero in almost all of the tissue which was regenerating, to increase the PCO_2 to levels in excess of 100 mm Hg, to depress the extracellular pH to below 6.8, and to raise the extracellular pK. Macrophages appeared to be able to resist an intracellular pH on the order of 5.7 or less without disintegration, but most other cells, including fibroblasts, began to show a loss of membrane potential and mitochondrial disruption when the intracellular pH dropped below 6.6. Loss of membrane potential was accompanied by sodium uptake due to the failure of the "sodium pump." This failure could be observed with "sodium" microelectrodes placed intracellularly or by "potassium" electrodes placed extracellularly, since failure of the sodium pump allowed the leakage of potassium out of the cells to balance the sodium which diffused into them. When cells were subjected to these conditions the mitochondria began to swell and, eventually, irreparable damage occurred, which was easily detectable at the ultrastructural level (Mela et al. 1972). Where this happened on a large scale, replenishment of the cell population either from elsewhere or from local cell division was necessary before healing could restart; but there is still considerable controversy as to the origin of these replacements (Büchner et al. 1970; Ross et al. 1970; Chapter 1, this volume). Another feature of hypoperfusion was the almost total extraction of glucose from the capillaries that were still open.

Effects of Infection

When organisms were introduced into a wound, they themselves modified the environment to a considerable extent. Aerobic bacteria frequently have a high oxygen consumption, especially when they are in the log phase of development (Smith et al. 1960; Bullen et al. 1966). This could be detected during the development of infection if microelectrodes were placed in the wound cavity or near the wound edge. Characteristic changes which accompany inflammation could be observed. As bacterial growth developed there was a fall in PO_2 in the wound dead space, but there was an early rise in PO_2 in the wound tissue which was apparently resulted from the poisoning of the cells in this area and reduction in their oxygen uptake together with the vasodilatation and increase in blood flow of the early inflammatory reaction. This was rapidly followed by a fall in PO_2 which appeared to be the result of both the increase in activity of neutrophil polymorphs of the "cellular phase" of inflammation and the oxygen uptake of the bacteria themselves. Finally, if the infection overwhelmed the local cellular defenses and the bacterial numbers increased, the oxygen tension fell to zero in the tissue as well as in the dead space.

Epithelial Regeneration

Epithelium migrating across an open wound is largely dependent for its energy supply under normal conditions on glycogen stored in the cells before migration takes place. Measurements under scabs in humans and in experimental animals (Silver 1972) have shown that the environmental conditions for the epithelial cells are relatively hostile. The oxygen tension is as low as might be predicted from a knowledge of the cellular environment at the edge of a wound. The normal dry scab is relatively impermeable to oxygen and the potential O_2 uptake of the epithelial cells is high. However, if epithelium is covered and kept moist by an oxygen-permeable membrane rather than by a dry scab, the rates of mitosis and migration are greatly increased (Hinman and Maibach 1963; Winter 1972). Epithelium does not appear to show any inhibition of mitosis or migration in oxygen tensions up to 700 mm Hg whereas fibroblasts do not grow satisfactorily if the oxygen tension rises about above 200 mm Hg (Niinikoski 1969).

In open wounds the oxygen supply to growing epithelium comes mostly from the atmosphere and to a very limited extent from the underlying connective tissue. The blood-borne supply is presumably limited because it reaches the epithelium in the face of competition from regenerating fibroblasts. The supply from the air is limited because of the relative impermeability of the scab and, therefore, epithelial aerobic respiration during migration and division must of necessity be restricted. Nevertheless, normal epithelium has the capacity for aerobic metabolism, and any system that can be devised for increasing the supply of oxygen, whether from the tissue or the atmosphere, is likely to encourage epithelial growth and migration. The chances of increasing the supply from the tissue are very limited because it has been found that when oxygen is given to a patient or to an experimental animal the rise PO_2 in the wound cavity is extremely small (Hunt et al. 1969; Silver 1969) since the fibroblasts covering the perfused capillaries in the wound edge are capable of taking up more oxygen than they normally obtain. In addition, giving oxygen for breathing usually results in peripheral vasoconstriction owing to the direct effect of high oxygen tension on capillary vessels. Thus, the administration of oxygen centrally is not a particularly effective way of raising the oxygen supply to the epithelium of a wound. In contrast to this, supplying oxygen locally by increasing the oxygen concentration of the atmosphere over a wound does have an obvious effect on epithelial and macrophage activity, if not on fibroblast proliferation and synthesis.

DISCUSSION

Wound repair ultimately requires that the conditions in the damaged area be favorable for the growth of fibroblasts, endothelial cells, and epithelium. From measurements of the conditions in wounds it seems that the natural state may represent a compromise which is evolutionarily successful but is not ideal for rapid healing and that this situation may be improved marginally by supplying extra oxygen locally. It is probably even more vital to insure that adequate circulation is available. This, of course, has been appreciated in surgical circles for a very long time. The importance of hypovolemia and of the overtreatment of shock must also be emphasized since it is perhaps not readily appreciated how sensitive new capillaries are to very small changes in the osmolarity or pressure of the blood, or how easily they leak when overfilled and close when under perfused. Factors such as circulating antibodies to substances like collagen, which may be released during trauma, especially burn trauma (Quismorio et al. 1971; Bray et al. 1969), may have a significant role in the slow healing response that is seen in burn injuries. Anticollagens could well act by "fixing" the protocollagen gel which is secreted by young fibroblasts and is utilized by growing endothelium to form a network of fibers around itself to support the newly canalized vessels and prevent them from being ruptured by blood pressure. In the absence of available protocollagen gel or where cross-linking is prevented as, for instance, in scurvy, bizarre forms of endothelial proliferation are seen, which lack support and tend to rupture when they become canalized.

The basic problem remains as to what is the stimulus for effective healing and what is the controlling mechanism which stops proliferation when a wound is filled with new tissue. If one observes the behavior of endothelial buds it is clear that they normally grow towards areas of low oxygen tension, but they will not do so unless they have been preceded by macrophage invasion. This applies both to the reorganization of blood supply around a foreign body in tissue and to the invasion of wound spaces. Maybe the endothelial cells can detect oxygen gradients and grow down them, but it is difficult to see how they can do this when they are growing from reasonably well-perfused normal tissue. Possibly the macrophage which has invaded the foreign body or the dead space in some way passes back a message to the endothelium. Perhaps the macrophage releases a substance during its phagocytic activity which provides a chemotaxic gradient for endothelium to follow. Maybe, as has been shown for antibody-producing lymphocytes, the macrophage processes the debris, moves back to the endothelial region, and passes a message in coded form to the endothelium which encourages it to grow in a particular direction into the new region. It is more certain that the macrophage can change the synthetic activity of fibroblasts, and perhaps other blood elements may be involved as well (see Chapters 1 and 22).

Whatever the mechanism which triggers the healing process, it is ultimately clear that the control of the local environment is dependent on the blood supply on the one hand and diffusion from the atmosphere on the other. It is also apparent that the proliferation of epithelium and of fibroblasts is to a large extent dependent on the oxygen microenvironment and to a lesser extent on the pH changes that occur in the tissue. Any form of treatment that encourages an increase of oxygen and reduces the time during which the wound is nonperfused will tend to increase the rate of healing.

ACKNOWLEDGMENTS

I am indebted to Mrs. Rachel Yerbury and Mr. C. Drown for invaluable technical assistance. Parts of this work were supported by U.S. government funds under contract DAJA-72-C-0962 and by NINDS Grant PO1 10939-03.

REFERENCES

Abercrombie M: Localised formation of new tissue in an adult mammal. Symp Soc Exp Biol 11:235, 1957

Baumgärtl H, Lübbers DW: Platinum needle electrode for polarographic measurement of oxygen and hydrogen. In Kessler M. et al. (eds.): Oxygen Supply. Munich, Urban und Schwarzenberg, 1973

Bray JP, Estess F, Bass JA: Anticollagen antibodies following thermal trauma. Proc Soc Exp Biol Med 130:394, 1969

Büchner T, Junge-Hülsing G, Wagner H, Oberwittler W, Hauss WH: Origin and formation of inflammatory cells in granulation tissue: Autoradiographic investigation with Thymidine-^{3}H on cotton pellet granuloma of the rat. Klin Wochenschr 48:867, 1970

Bullen JJ, Cushnie GH, Stoner HB: Oxygen uptake by Clostridium welchii type A: Its possible role in experimental infections in passively immunised animals. Br J Exp Pathol 47:488, 1966

Bullough WS: Mitotic and functional homeostasis: A speculative review. Cancer Res 25:1683, 1965

Bullough WS: The actions of chalones. Agents Actions 2:1, 1971

Bullough WS, Lawrence EB: The diurnal cycle in epidermal mitotic duration and its relation to chalone and adrenalin. Exp Cell Res 43:343, 1966

Bullough WS, Lawrence EB: Control of mitosis in mouse and hamster melanomata by means of the melanocytes chalone. Eur J Cancer 4:607, 1968

Bullough WS, Lawrence EB: The lymphatic chalone and its antimitotic action on a mouse lymphoma in vitro. Eur J Cancer 6:525, 1970

Clark R, Stone RD, Leung DYK, Silver IA, Hohn D, Hunt TK: Role of macrophages in wound healing. Surg Forum 27:16, 1976

Cross JP: A technique for the assay of granulocyte chalone and antichalone. J Anat 111:336, 1972

Gabbiani G, Majno G, Ryan GB: The fibroblast as a contractile cell: The myofibroblast. In Kulonen E, Pikkarainen, J (eds): The Biology of the Fibroblast. London, Academic Press, 1973

Hell EA: Stimulatnts to D.N.A. synthesis in guinea pig ear epidermis. Br J Dermatol 83:632, 1970

Hinman CD, Maibach H: Effects of air exposure and occlusion on experimental human skin wounds. Nature 200:377, 1963

Hunt TK, Hutchison JGP: Studies on oxygen tension in healing wounds. In Illingworth CF (ed): Wound Healing. London, Churchill, 1966

Hunt TK, Zederfeldt B: Nutritional and environmental aspects of wound healing. In Dunphy JE, Van Winkle W (eds): Repair and Regeneration. New York, McGraw-Hill, 1969

Hunt TK, Twomey P, Zederfeldt B, Dunphy JE: Respiratory gas tensions and pH in healing wounds. Amer J Surg 114:302, 1967

Hunt TK, Zederfeldt B, Dunphy JE: The role of oxygen tension in healing. J Surg, (Banares, Hindu Univ) 4:279, 1968

Hunt TK, Zederfeldt B, Goldstick TK: Oxygen and healing. Amer J Surg 118:521, 1969

Kulonen E, Niinikoski J: Effect of hyberbaric oxygenation on wound healing and experimental granulomata. Acta Physiol Scand 73:383, 1968

Lübbers DW, Baumgärtl H: Herstellungstechnik von palladinierten Pt-stichelectroden (1-5μ aussendurchmesser) zur polarographischen messung des wasserstoffdruckes fur die bestimmung der mikrozirkulation. Pflugers Arch 294, R.39, 1967

Marks R: The role of chalones in epidermal homeostasis. Br J Dermatol 86:543, 1972

Maroudas A: Discussion. Philos Trans R Soc Lond [Biol] 271, 272, 1975

Mela LM, Miller LD, Nicholas GG: Influence of cellular acidosis and altered cation concentrations on shock-induced mitochondrial damage. Surgery 72:102, 1972

Niinikoski J: Effect of oxygen supply on wound healing and formation of experimental granulation tissue. Acta Physiol Scand [Suppl] 334:74, 1969

Niinikoski J, Kulonen E: Reparation at increased oxygen supply. Experientia 26:247, 1970

Ordman LJ, Gillman T: Studies on the healing of cutaneous wounds. 1. The healing of incisions through the skin of pigs. Arch Surg 83:857, 1966a

Ordman LJ, Gillman T: Studies on the healing of cutaneous wounds. 2. The healing of epidermal, appendageal and dermal injuries inflicted by suture needles and by the suture material in the skin of pigs. Arch Surg 93:883, 1966b

Ordman LJ, Gillman T: Studies on the healing of cutaneous wounds. 3. A critical comparison in the pig of the healing of surgical incisions closed with sutures or adhesive tape, based on tensile strength, and clinical and histological criteria. Arch Surg 93:911, 1966c

Quismorio FB, Bland SL, Frion GJ: Autoimmunity in thermal injury. Clin Exp Immunol 8:701, 1971

Remensnyder JP, Majno G: Oxygen gradients in healing wounds. Amer J Pathol 52:301, 1968

Ross R, Everett NB, Tyler R: Wound healing and collagen formation: VI. Origin of wound fibroblasts studied in parabiosis. J Cell Biol 44:645, 1970

Silver IA: Some observations on the cerebral cortex with an ultramicro, membrane covered oxygen electrode. Med Electron Biol Engng 3:377, 1965

Silver IA: The measurement of oxygen tension in living tissue. In Payne JP, Hill DW (eds): Oxygen Measurements in Blood and Tissues. London, Churchill, 1966

Silver IA: The measurement of oxygen tension in healing tissue. Prog Resp Res 3:124, 1969

Silver IA: Oxygen tension and epithelialization. In Maibach HI, Rovee DT (eds): Epidermal Wound Healing. Chicago, Year Book, 1972

Silver IA: Some problems in the investigation of tissue micro-environment. Adv Chem 118:343, 1973a

Silver IA: Local and systemic factors which affect the proliferation of fibroblasts. In Kulonen E, Pikkareinen J (eds): The Biology of the Fibroblast. London, Academic Press, 1973b

Silver IA: Ionic composition of pericellular sites. Philos Trans Soc Lond [Biol] 271:261, 1975

Silver IA: A microglucose electrode. In Kessler M et al (eds): Ion Selective and Enzyme Electrodes in Biology and Medicine. Munich, Urban und Schwarzenberg, 1976

Smith IM, Wilson, AP, Hazard EC, Hummer WK, Dewey ME: Studies on the mechanism of death of mice infected with staphylococci. Infect Dis 107:369, 1960

Thomas RC: New design for a sodium sensitive glass microelectrode. J Physiol (Lond) 210:82P, 1970

Thomas RC: Construction and properties of recessed-tip microelectrodes for Na+, pH and Cl−. In Kessler M et al. (eds): Ion Selective and Enzyme Microelectrodes in Biology and Medicine. Munich, Urban und Schwarzenberg, 1976

Winter G: Epidermal regeneration studies in the domestic pig. In Maibach HI, Rovee DT (eds): Epidermal Wound Healing. Chicago, Year Book, 1972

Wood S, Lewis R, Mulholland JH, Knaack J: Assembly, insertion and use of a modified rabbit ear chamber. Bull Johns Hopkins Hosp 119:1, 1966

Zeuthen T, Hiam RC, Silver IA: Recording of ion activities in the brain. In Berman H, Herbert N (eds): Ion Selective Microelectrodes. New York, Plenum Press, 1974

Comment

I wish that this superb essay could be read by every surgeon. Dr. Silver modestly gives credit for environmental studies to others in his introduction and then demonstrates his mastery of the field in the rest of the essay.

In a number of conversations, Dr. Silver and I have conceived the idea of the "module" of reparative tissue. Perhaps he is not as attracted to it as I am, or he might have included it in the essay. Perhaps he wants me to explain it. Figure 6 is a schematic drawing of an ear chamber wound at right angles to the diagrams shown by Dr. Silver. The module is centered about a blood vessel which is budding to supply the advancing cells in response to a signal coming from that area. The macrophage in the van ahead of it is guiding the way and probably orchestrating the events which follow (see Chapter 1). The fibroblast is the third and last major cellular component. Other neutrophiles are there—but mainly to resist infection. The ecology of the module strikingly demonstrates the interdependence of these cells and structures. Fibroblasts and their collagen provide support for the macrophage, the endothelial bud, and the completed vessel. But fibroblasts probably can't multiply without the macrophage and can't produce collagen without nutrient supply from the vessel, and the vessel can't withstand its internal blood pressure without collagenous support. Thus, the module, or "cell team," proceeds across the wound space with none of its components able to act alone.

With this in mind, it is interesting to reflect on the scirrhous breast cancer. Antigens to malignant cells combine with receptors on macrophages, presumably "activating" them. Dense connective-tissue and blood-vessel ingrowth occurs, though in this tumor example tumor-angiogenetic stimulators may also play a role. This macrophagic mechanism probably applies to rheumatoid arthritis, tuberculosis, and others without aid of tumor-originated stimuli.

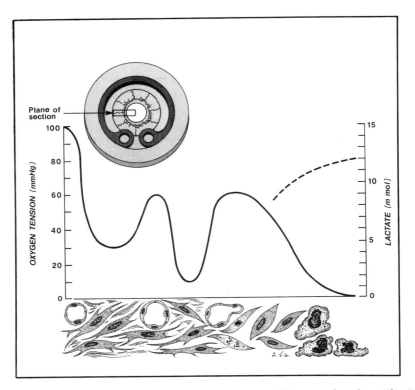

FIG 6.   *Side view of the wound module as in a rabbit ear chamber. The Po₂ profile is shown above the tissue. Note the peaks over the vessels and the long gradient down to almost zero at the wound edge. Note the lactate gradient, high in the dead space and lower towards the vasculature. This demonstrates how the central wound remains hypoxic and acidotic despite the advancing vasculature. (Hunt TK, Dunphy JE (eds): Fundamentals of Wound Management, p. 55. Copyright © 1979 Appleton-Century-Crofts. Prepared in cooperation with Dr. I. A. Silver)*

As we will show later, products of clotting can activate macrophages, and with platelet factor(s) are probably the earliest signals for repair. This tends to confirm Dr. Silver's observation that the macrophage seems to ingest and digest the blood clot before replacing it. (The module concept than may explain the revascularization of thrombosed veins.)

His comments on hypovolemia should be emphasized by translation to surgical language. Every surgeon knows that ischemic tissue heals poorly and becomes infected. As surgeons, we have assumed that there is a point of vascularity at which this ceases to be true. His observations (and mine) show that there is no such *point*. Each decrement of oxygen availablity takes its toll—starting from normal!

Dr. Silver has introduced, for its first time in this book, the concept of Gabbiani et al. (1972) who, in investigating wound contraction, first demonstrated myofibrils in cells which otherwise appear to be fibroblasts. Earlier, James et al. (reviewed in Montandon et al. 1977) measured the force of contraction and showed that it is in the range of that developed by smooth muscle cells. Since then, others (e.g., Guber and Rudolph 1978) have seen these cells in wounds, atheromatous vessels, etc. They can contract, and they behave like smooth muscle when stimulated with acetylcholine or relaxed with atropine. They also synthesize collagen and appear to be the native force of wound contraction.

Dr. Silver is not primarily a "wound healer." However, he has such a mastery of the ear-chamber technique and oxygen-measuring devices that he is, perhaps, the researcher most intimately acquainted with the physiology of the normal healing wound in all its moods. Certainly, he is the world's expert on the microcirculation in repair.

REFERENCES

Gabbiani G, Hirschel BJ, Ryan GB, et al.: Granulation tissue as a contractive organ. A study of structure and function. J Exp Med 135:719, 1972

Guber S, Rudolph R: The myofibroblast. Surg Gynecol Obstet 146:641, 1978

Montandon D, D'Andiran G, Gabbiani G: The mechanism of wound contraction and epithelization. Clinical and experimental studies. Clin Plast Surg 4: 325, 1977

The Biochemical Basis of Repair
3

D. S. Jackson

The tensile strength and the collagen content of an incised wound show a parallel increase particularly during the middle phase, i.e., between the fifth and fifteenth days. Prior to the fifth day the tensile strength and the collagen content are low. The early events taking place during these first five days are clearly of considerable importance as is made clear by other papers in this volume. Essentially, they insure that a colony of fully functioning fibroblasts is established in the wound, where they proceed to lay down a predominantly collagen structure to fill the defect created by the wound.

The structures of the connective tissues are based on essentially the same macromolecules: collagen, elastin, proteoglycans, and glycoproteins. Nevertheless, a wide variety of connective tissues with widely differing structures and functions are found in nature. Some of these differences may be found in the variations in amounts of elastin, proteoglycans, and glycoproteins associated with collagen, but since collagen constitutes the bulk of many connective tissues it must make a major contribution to their properties. For example, although collagen accounts for over 80 percent of the dry weight of tendon, skin, and cornea, the architecture and function of these tissues are quite different. As described in Chapter 10, the architecture of the dermal scar tissue is considerably different from that of dermis, and it never functions as efficiently in its mechanical properties, despite the fact that scar collagen is not unlike that of the dermis and that both structures have a similar collagen content.

The collagen molecules in all tissues are essentially the same but there are subtle variations on the basic theme which may play a part in determining biological function. In this chapter I discuss the general pattern of collagen structure and biosynthesis and then deal with more specific aspects of scar collagen and the differences between that and dermal collagen, which may account for some of the strucutral and functional differences.

COLLAGEN STRUCTURE

All extracellular collagens so far investigated consist of three polypeptide chains (α-chains) which are wound around each other to form a special type of helix. Unusual features are the presence of hydroxyproline and hydroxylysine, both of which have important roles in defining the final fiber structure. A number of the hydroxylysine residues have sugars attached to them, these glycosyl residues being linked through the hydroxyl group. The overall picture of the collagen molecule (tropocollagen) is of a long, thin, fairly rigid rod approximately 290×1.4 nm which can spontaneously aggregate into fibrils of the kind seen by electron microscopy in most connective tissues. These aggregates are stabilized by covalent cross-links and it is these which give the fibrils the tensile strength which is so important in the surgical wound.

VARIATION ON THE BASIC THEME

Genetic Polymorphism

In recent years it has become apparent that the cells of higher organisms contain several different structural genes directing collagen synthesis. Five different types of α-chains have been identified in vertebrate tissues, which give rise to four different collagen types. As can be seen in Table 1 there is some degree of specificity in the type of collagen found in various tissues, indicating the selectivity of gene expression for collagen biosynthesis in certain cell types.

In tissues such as bone, tendon, mature dermis, cornea, and sclera, the chain composition is $[\alpha 1(I)]_2 \alpha 2$, i.e., having two identical chains $\alpha 1(I)$, the third member of the triple helix having a different primary structure, $\alpha 2$, and the complete molecule being referred to as Type I collagen. The major collagen type in cartilage is Type II, which has three identical α-chains of different primary structure to $\alpha 1(I)$ and designated $\alpha 1(II)$, with the chain composition $[\alpha 1(II)]_3$. Yet another type of interstitial collagen has been found and named Type III. It too has three identical α-chains of unique primary structure, the molecule

Table 1. Collagen Polymorphism in Various Tissues

Type	Molecular Form	Tissue
I	$[\alpha 1(I)]_2\alpha 2$	Bone, dermis, tendon, cornea, dentin
II	$[\alpha 1(II)]_3$	Cartilages
III	$[\alpha 1(III)]_3$	Fetal and infant dermis, cardiovascular system
IV	$[\alpha 1(IV)]_3$	Basement membranes

*Tissues mentioned contain predominantly the collagen type indicated, but many tissues have been found to contain more than one collagen type.

Table 2. Variations in the Contents of Hydroxyproline, Hydroxylysine, and Hydroxylysine Glycosides in Several Vertebrate Collagens

	Hydroxyproline*		Hydroxy-lysine	Substituted Hydroxy-lysine	Distribution of Carbohydrate Units (%)	
	4-isomer	3-isomer			Hyl-Gal	Hyl-Gal-Glc
Type I						
Human sclera	88.6		6.4	1.7	30	70
Human dermis	92.1		3.6	1.4	30	70
Human tendon	85.9		8.7	1.4	40	60
Human cornea	82.9		8.7	6.4	30	70
Type II						
Chick cartilage	103	2	23	9.2	40	60
Type III						
Human aorta	125		5			
Type IV						
Human glomerular basement membrane	130	11	45	36	5	95
Bovine anterior lens capsule	132	10	57	42	3	97

*Data in residues/1000.

Table 3. Cross-link Patterns of Various Tissues

Cross-link	Tissues
Hydroxylysinonorleucine	Adult skin
Hydroxylysinonorleucine and hydroxylysinohydroxynorleucine	Tendon, cornea, lens capsule, kidney glomerulus, intervertebral disc
Hydroxylysinohydroxynorleucine	Bone, cartilage, cardiac tendon, uterus, scar, embryonic skin

being designated [α1(III)]$_3$. This collagen is also unusual in that it contains cysteine and is disulphide bonded. This type of collagen was first found in embryonic dermis. Postnatally there is a switch from Type III to Type I synthesis, with the result that the bulk of the collagen in adult dermis is Type I. Type III also occurs in cardiovascular tissues, constituting, for example, some 50 percent of the collagen of the human aorta.

A class of connective tissues distinct from others is found in the basement membrane. From these a further type of collagen (Type IV) has been isolated and characterized. This has three identical α-chains [(α1)IV] of unique primary structure and is designated [(α1)IV]$_3$.

Secondary Modifications

Another kind of variation is found in the proportion of lysine residues that are hydroxylated to hydroxylysine and the degree of glycosylation of these hydroxylysines. The variations can occur within a given collagen type as well as between the different types (Table 2). Thus, tendon collagen, which is Type I, has 4 to 6 residues of hydroxylysine and only 2 carbohydrate molecules, compared to corneal collagen, also Type I, which has 10 residues of each. There are also differences to be found in the relative proportions of Hyl-Gal and Hyl-Gal-Glc.

A further modification is the formation of covalent cross-links involving lysine and hydroxylysine in the terminal residues. Two different types of cross-links are known, and as can be seen from Table 3 these too are a source of variability of collagen structure.

These variations in primary structure and in secondary modification can clearly give rise to quite a large number of distinctive collagen molecules, each of which could possibly result in the formation of fibrous structures with different architectural arrangements and, hence, of different properties and functions.

BIOSYNTHESIS OF PROCOLLAGEN

Synthesis of Primary Structure (pro-α-chains)

As initially synthesized the polypeptide chains are significantly larger than the extracellular tropocollagen α-chains. The increase in size is due to the presence of peptides (which are nonhelical) at the end of the molecule with molecular weights of 15,000 to 20,000 and 33,000 to 37,000 daltons respectively. These precursor chains (with the terminal peptides attached) named pro-α-chains, also differ from tropocollagen in that they contain cysteine.

Hydroxylation

The amino acids hydroxyproline and hydroxylysine, characteristic of all collagens, are absent from the pro-α-chains when initially synthesized. Specific proline and lysine residues are hydroxylated by prolyl and lysyl hydroxylases both of which require Fe^{++}, α-ketoglutarate, O_2, and ascorbic acid as cofactors. These enzymes are bound to the rough endoplasmic reticulum and the hydroxylation commences on nascent polypeptide chains attached to membrane-bound ribosomes.

Glycosylation

All vertebrate collagens contain glucose and galactose linked through the hydroxyl group of hydroxylsine residues and, hence, glycosylation is subsequent to hydroxylation. The two hexoses are found as galactosyl hydroxylysine or glucosyl-galactosyl hydroxylysine. Galactosyl and glucosyl transferases are involved, galactose being first attached to hydroxylysine and glucose being attached to the galactosyl hydroxylysine to form a disaccharide. Both enzymes are membrane bound, largely to the rough endoplasmic reticulum but with a significant proportion bound to the smooth endoplasmic reticulum.

Formation of Interchain Disulphide Bonds and the Triple Helix

Unlike extracellular Type I and Type II tropocollagen, the corresponding procollagens contain cysteine residues located in the N-terminal region. Procollagen is secreted by cultured cells in a triple helical conformation that contains interchain disulphide bonds. Recent evidence indicates that soon after the pro-α-chains are released from the ribosomes into the cisternae of the endoplasmic reticulum interchain disulphide bonds are formed and the triple-helical conformation rapidly assumed by the pro-α-chains. This assembly of pro-α-chains apparently begins in the cisternae of rough endoplasmic reticulum and is completed in the cisternae of smooth endoplasmic reticulum.

The whole process is summarized in Figure 1, which illustrates the intracellular pathway taken by the procollagen, beginning with its synthesis on the membrane-bound ribosomes. This is followed by successive hydroxylation and glycosylation as the polypeptide chain peels off the ribosome into the cisternae of the endoplasmic reticulum where the completed pro-α-chains align themselves in register, allowing disulphide bonds to form and the polypeptide chains to take up the triple-helical conformation.

The types of collagen appear to differ in the time required for synthesis and secretion, Type I taking the shortest time and Type IV the

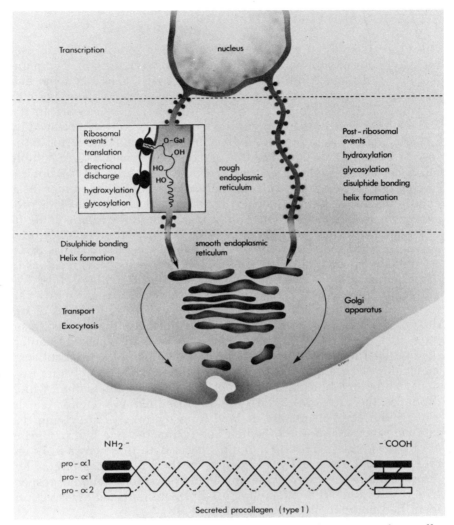

FIG. 1. Schematic representation of the synthesis and secretion of procollagen. (Grant ME, Jackson DS. In Campbell PH, Aldridge WN (eds): Essays in
Biochemistry, vol 12. Copyright © 1976 Academic Press)

longest. The time of formation of the triple helix follows the same
pattern; and, since hydroxylation and glycosylation can only occur
while the pro-α-chains are in a random-coil configuration, these time
differences may be important in deciding the degree of hydroxylation
and glycosylation that takes place.

SECRETION AND FIBRIL FORMATION

Once the assembly of procollagen molecules is complete they are secreted via the smooth endoplasmic reticulum, including the Golgi apparatus, and thence into the extracellular space. There is some evidence that the procollagen is packaged into membrane-bound vesicles in which it is transported to the cell surface and released into the extracellular space. At this point the terminal peptides are cleaved by specific peptidases to produce extracellular tropocollagen. Prior to the loss of the terminal peptides, the procollagen molecules are soluble under certain physiological conditions of temperature and pH, but following this loss the tropocollagen molecules are insoluble under these conditions and can spontaneously combine and precipitate. This process is analogous to the formation of insoluble fibrin from soluble fibrinogen. One further modification also takes place in the extracellular space, i.e., the formation of the precursors of the stabilizing cross-links. An oxidative deamination of specific lysyl or hydroxylysyl residues in the terminal regions occurs, involving an amino oxidase which requires Cu^{++} as a cofactor. The products are aldehyde groups which can react spontaneously with the ϵ-NH_2 groups of adjacent lysines or hydroxylysines to form covalent cross-links. Initially, the tropocollagen molecules aggregate by a self-assembly process in a specific conformation determined by the charge distribution along the tropocollagen molecules. This alignment brings the lysine and hydroxylysine residues in adjacent molecules into a position allowing interaction, which produces the cross-links. Two major cross-links are found: one in which both components are derived from hydroxylysine, giving rise to a keto-imine, and one in which one lysine and one hydroxylysine are involved, giving rise to a Schiff's base. Both these cross-links are reducible and are usually designated by their reduced products hydroxylysinohydroxynorleucine and hydroxylysinonorleucine, respectively. With time, the reducible cross-links are replaced by as yet unidentified nonreducible compounds.

SPECIFIC ASPECTS OF SCAR COLLAGEN

Genetic Type

Collagen from guinea pig scar was found to be Type I (Shuttleworth and Forrest 1974) and wound tissue *in vitro* synthesized only Type I (Shuttleworth et al, 1975). It has been reported, however, that normal human scars (Epstein and Munderloh 1975), hypertrophic scars (Epstein and Munderloh 1975, Bailey et al. 1975a), and keloid (Epstein and Munderloh 1975) contain a large proportion of Type III collagen. This is also true of granulation tissue formed in response to acute inflammation by turpentine injection or to chronic inflammation by sponge implantation (Bailey et al. 1975b). The normal adult dermis contains a low proportion of Type III, and the presence of Type III in human scars could affect the tensile strength of fibers in the wounds and could be one reason for the differences found between the tensile strength of wounds and dermis.

Secondary Modifications

Table 2 shows that scar collagen differs from dermal collagen in both hydroxylysine and hexose content. There are 8 residues of hydroxy-lysine and 10 residues of hexose compared with 4 and 2, respectively, in dermal collagen. Much of the increase in carbohydrate results from the higher proportion of disaccharide units found in scar collagen.

Guinea pig scar collagen contains largely the cross-links derived from hydroxyallysine and hydroxylysine whereas dermal collagen contains cross-links derived from allysine. This is probably due to the greater degree of hydroxylation in scar collagen of the N-terminal lys-ine involved in cross-link formation. In human scar collagen, however, this pattern changes as time passes towards the dermal pattern. The same shift from dihydroxylysinonorleucine to hydroxylysinonorleu-cine is seen in the dermis postnatally and may be part of a general development from embryonic to mature tissue.

Interaction with Noncollagenous Components

Dermal insoluble collagen can be readily purified either by extraction with EDTA or by treatment with a crude bacterial α-amylase. The hexosamine content of this preparation is barely measureable and the hexose content can be accounted for by the glucose and galactose residues attached to collagen through hydroxylysine. Following such treatment, dermal collagen is readily dispersible in dilute acetic acid.

In contrast, scar collagen treated with these reagents contains hexosamine and more carbohydrate than can be accounted for by glycosylated hydroxylysine. Further, the glycine content is low and there are differences in the number of residues of other amino acids as compared with those in dermal collagen. These analytical differences indicate the presence of a firmly bound glycoprotein not present in purified dermal collagen. The scar collagen was not dispersible in dilute acetic acid which suggests that the glycoprotein acts as a kind of cement substance holding together scar collagen fibrils.

STRUCTURE AND FUNCTION RELATIONSHIPS

The physical properties of skin wounds are significantly different from those of intact skin. Although the strength of scar increases steadily over a long period of time, the tensile strength fails to reach that of intact skin, and the scar is also less elastic. The scar collagen has thinner fibrils and lacks the well-defined architecture seen in the normal dermis, the fibers being coarse, irregular, and arranged somewhat randomly. In the guinea pig, over a period of some four weeks, the diameter of the fibrils in the scar changes from having a median of 80 nm with a range of 40 to 1000 nm to a median of 50 nm with a much narrower range. This may be related to the hexose content of the collagen, which is similar to that found in cornea which is also characterized by small-diameter fibrils with small variation.

At the biochemical level we have seen that the scar collagen has a collagen polymorphism not found in dermis, having both Type I and Type III present. It differs in its degree of the hydroxylation of lysine and the glycosylation of hydroxylysine. The cross-linking pattern is different, although the scar pattern does eventually change towards the dermal pattern. There is also the more firm interaction between scar collagen and a noncollagenous matrix. All of these differences may lead directly to the differences in structure and function between scar and dermal tissue or may be responsible for the different architecture which in itself has different structural and mechanical properties.

ABNORMAL SCAR FORMATION

The detailed knowledge we now possess of collagen structure and biosynthesis enables us to carry out more detailed and refined studies of the normal wound-healing process and also of those leading to abnormal scar-tissue formation. Recent studies have shown that the rate of biosynthesis of hypertrophic and keloid scar collagen is initially about twice the rate of that of normal scar collagen. It is little different, however, from that found in normal dermis, and after two or three years it falls to the level of normal scar. Prolyl hydroxylase levels are higher than those found in normal scar and dermis. Since there is an obvious accumulation of scar tissue in these two pathological conditions, the absence of any really marked difference in the rate of collagen synthesis suggested a failure of resorption. However, the levels of the enzyme collagenase thought to be responsible for degradation of collagen are also quite similar in both normal and pathological tissues, but the method of measurement, i.e., *in vitro* incubation, may lead to a nonspecific activation of the known zymogen precursor of collagenase. There is some evidence that the normal activating system is defective in keloid. There is also evidence of high concentrations of collagenase inhibitors, α_1-antitrypsin and α_2-macroglobulin in keloid and hypertrophic scars.

REFERENCES

Bailey AJ, Robins SP, Balian G: Biological significance of the intermolecular crosslink of collagen. Nature 251:105, 1974

Bailey AJ, Sims TJ, Le Lous M, Bazin S: Collagen polymorphism in experimental granulation tissues. Biochem Biophys Res Commun 66: 1160, 1975b

Bailey AJ, Bazin S, Sims TJ, Le Lous M, Nicoletis C, Delaunay A: Characterisation of the collagen of human hypertrophic and normal scars. Biochim Biophys Acta 405: 412, 1975a

Epstein EH Jr, Munderloh NH: Isolation and characterisation of CNBr peptides of human Type III collagen and tissue distributary Type I and Type III collagen. J Biol Chem 250: 9304, 1975

Shuttleworth CA, Forrest L: Pepsin-solubilized collagen of guinea pig dermis and dermal scar. Biochim Biophys Acta 365: 454, 1974

Shuttleworth CA, Forrest L, Jackson DS: Comparison of cyanogen bromide peptides of insoluble guinea-pig skin and scar collagen. Biochim Biphys Acta 379: 207, 1975

GENERAL REFERENCES

Grant ME, Jackson DS: The biosynthesis of procollagen, In Campbell PN, Aldridge WN (eds): Essays in Biochemistry, vol. 12, New York, Academic Press, 1976

Van der Meulen JC (ed): First International Symposium on Wound Healing 1974. Proceedings. Montreux, Foundation for International Cooperation in the Medical Sciences, 1974

Prockup DJ, Berg RA, Kivirikko KI, Uitto J: Intracellular Steps in the Biosynthesis of Collagen. In Ramachandran GN, Reddi AH (eds): Biochemistry of Collagen, New York, Plenum Press, 1976

Comment

This essay summarizes almost everything the surgeon needs to know about collagen, and then some. There are several important conclusions: the healing wound has a different collagenous pattern than its host tissue and, although the chemical variations are not exactly the same in bone, differences between healing bone and normal bone also exist. Furthermore, as Dr. Forrester (Chapter 10) will also point out, scar collagen is not only chemically different, it is morphologically different as well.

To help those who may be bewildered by the terminology, the following may be helpful.

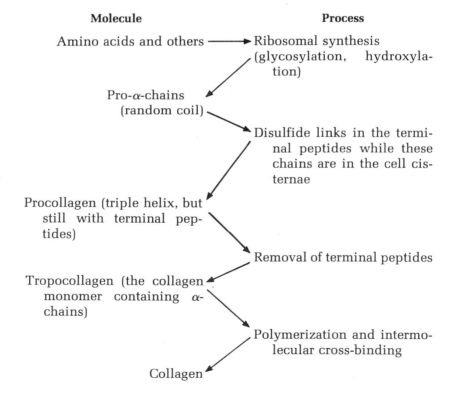

Molecule   **Process**

Amino acids and others ⟶ Ribosomal synthesis (glycosylation, hydroxylation)

Pro-α-chains (random coil)

Disulfide links in the terminal peptides while these chains are in the cell cisternae

Procollagen (triple helix, but still with terminal peptides)

Removal of terminal peptides

Tropocollagen (the collagen monomer containing α-chains)

Polymerization and intermolecular cross-binding

Collagen

One of the key sentences of this chapter is the "the tensile strength . . . of scar . . . fails to reach that of intact skin, and the scar is also less elastic." One occasionally sees an athletic patient with a full-thickness burn who actually ruptures the burn scar during a vigorous movement. Boxers (at least the losers) know that once scar tissue is formed over the eye, the affected skin is fragile. And every surgeon who tries to repair an incisional hernia by closing scar to scar should know that such repairs tend to fail. The old saw that fractured bone is stronger than normal is not true.

As for hypertrophic scar and keloid, Dr. Jackson has skimmed away some of the film over very murky water. Collagen synthesis and lysis both seem to be somewhat elevated in each of these conditions, at least during the formative stages. To demonstrate the subtleties involved, however, it has been calculated that the difference between the normal slim person and the morbidly obese person, i.e., over 300 pounds, might be only the difference between eating one or two slices of bread a day over a period of years. When one takes into account that normal skin collagen turns over and that scar collagen turns over rather more rapidly for at least a year or two, one can see that in order to achieve twice the bulk of a normal area of skin, one need add (or retain) only a small amount of collagen at any given moment in order to make a large difference in the long run. The intimate secrets of keloid and hypertrophic scar remain hidden (Ketchum et al. 1974).

The concept of a balance of collagen synthesis and lysis in the healing wound has proved to be one of considerable surgical importance. While many of us have known for years that there had to be such a "balance," Dr. Jackson, with Kevin Cronin and J.E. Dunphy, was the first to point out how important it can be when they noted a lysis of as much as 50 percent of old collagen in the area of a rat colon anastomosis at one week after operation. Obviously, synthesis *must* make up this deficit or the suture line will fail. This concept is treated more extensively in Chapter 13. There has been some controversy over the actual extent of the lysis, but even the lowest estimated (about 25 percent loss in the first week) are large enough to emphasize the importance of the concept.

REFERENCE

Ketchum LD, Cohen IK, Master FW: Hypertrophic scars and keloids: A collective review. Plast Reconstr Surg 53:140, 1974

Proteoglycans of the Connective Tissue Ground Substance

4

J. Peter Bentley

The process of wound healing is usually accompanied by the filling of a defect with connective tissue and, indeed, this could possibly serve as a definition of wound healing. All connective tissues contain in varying amounts a component sometimes referred to as *ground substance*. This amorphous matrix between the cells and fibers contains a variety of serum proteins and salts, and, in addition, it contains high concentrations of a specific class of compounds collectively referred to as *connective tissue proteoglycans*. Several years ago, these substances were known as *acid mucopolysaccharides* because they are largely polysaccharide in nature and have a great affinity for the basic dyes used in histological preparations. During the 1960s, a new name was proposed for these compounds[1] and they became known as *glycosaminoglycuronoglycans* or, more briefly, *glycosaminoglycans*.* It was, of course, known that glycosaminoglycans were bound to protein, and for a while the term *protein polysaccharide complex* was used.

Today, the protein polysaccharide complexes of connective tissue are generally referred to as *proteoglycans*, which emphasizes their predominantly carbohydrate nature in contradistinction to glycoproteins, which consist mainly of protein and contain variable but relatively

---

Glycosaminoglycans are sometimes referred to as *mucopolysaccharides*. A group of polysaccharides composed of repeating disaccharide units of a hexosamine and a hexuronic acid (except keratan sulfate in which galactose replaces the hexuronic acid) linked by glycoside bonds. The amine group of the hexosamine usually is either N-acetylated or N-sulfated. See Table 1 for a list of repeating disaccharides of each glycosaminoglycan.

small amounts of attached carbohydrate. All connective tissues studied contain glycosaminoglycans presumably in the form of proteoglycans, but detailed structural analysis has been carried out only upon the proteoglycans of cartilage. The currently accepted model for cartilage proteoglycan is shown in Figure 1. It is composed of a central protein core with a molecular weight of approximately 200,000. This protein core appears to consist of three regions. There is a region in which chondroitin sulfate side chains predominate, and which contains relatively little keratan sulfate, and another region to which more than 50 percent of the keratan sulfate chains are attached. Yet a third region consisting of approximately 30 percent of the total protein core contains few, if any, polysaccharide chains, and this region is capable of interacting with and binding the entire proteoglycan to a molecule of hyaluronic acid.[2,3] The average molecular weight of the chondroitin sulfate side chains is about 20,000 and that of the keratan sulfate side chains is about 8,000, although there is considerable variability about these mean values.[3] The proteoglycan can be digested with general proteases, such as pronase or papain, which degrade the core protein and release free glycosaminoglycan side chains containing a few amino acids that were originally part of the protein core. If an entire tissue is

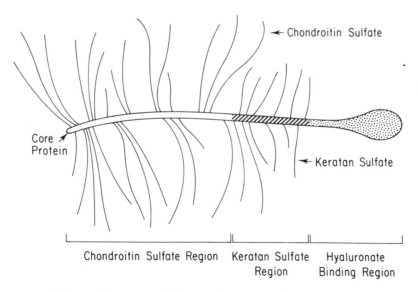

Core Protein

Chondroitin Sulfate

Keratan Sulfate

| Chondroitin Sulfate Region | Keratan Sulfate Region | Hyaluronate Binding Region |

FIG. 1. *Structure of the cartilage proteoglycans monomer.*

TABLE 1.   Glycosaminoglycan Composition

	Repeating Disaccharide	Location
Hyaluronic acid	Glucuronic acid (β 1→3) glucosamine	Embryonic tissues, synovial fluid, vitreous humor, umbilical cord, cartilage, early healing tissue (inflammatory phases)
Chondroitin-4-sulfate	Glucuronic acid (β 1→3) galactosamine-4-SO_4	Cartilage, skin, cornea, blood vessel wall, nucleus
Chondroitin-6-sulfate	Glucuronic acid (β 1→3) galactosamine-6-SO_4	pulposis, later healing (associated with collagen synthesis)
Dermatan sulfate	Iduronic acid (β 1→3) galactosamine-4-SO_4*	Skin, blood vessels, heart valves, umbilical cord, scar
Keratan sulfate	Galactose (β 1→4) glucosamine-6-SO_4	Cornea, cartilage, nucleus pulposis
Heparin and heparan sulfate	Glucuronic acid-2-SO_4 (1→4) glucosamine-2-SO_4 and -6-SO_4†	Many tissues in mast cells (heparin); universal cell surface component (heparan sulfate)

*Also contains glucuronic acid; some of the iduronates are 2-sulfated.

†Much variation in degree of sulfation; contains α- and β-links and some iduronate.

treated in this way, the glycosaminoglycan chains can be separated by several different techniques prior to chemical characterization. This type of analysis was carried out several years ago,[4] and it was noted that different tissues contained different complements of glycosaminoglycan, presumably (as pointed out above) bound in some form of proteoglycans. The various glycosaminoglycans consist of disaccharide repeating units, usually containing an amino sugar and a glucuronic acid. The repeating sequences of the glycosaminoglycans of connective tissue are shown in Table 1.

CARBOHYDRATE LINKAGE REGIONS

Chondroitin sulfate, dermatan sulfate, and heparin sulfate are covalently attached to the protein core at the reducing end of the molecule by a tetrasaccharide known as the linkage region, and the terminal sugar of this linkage region, xylose, is bound to serine in the protein core by an O-glycoside linkage. The linkage of keratan sulfate is somewhat different and appears to be a glycoside bond[*] between galacto-samine and serine and/or threonine. The galactosamine is substituted at position 3 with a neuraminyl-galactosyl disaccharide, and at position 6 with the keratan sulfate chain.[5] These linkage regions are shown schematically below.

$$\begin{bmatrix} \text{Chondroitin-SO}_4 \\ \text{or} \\ \text{Dermatan-SO}_4 \\ \text{or} \\ \text{Heparan-SO}_4 \end{bmatrix} \text{———} \; \text{GlcUA—Gal—Gal—Xyl—O—Ser} \begin{matrix} \{ \\ \\ \{ \end{matrix}$$

Keratan-SO$_4$
|
Sial—Gal—GalNAc—O—Ser (or Thr)

PROTEOGLYCAN AGGREGATION

Proteoglycans can best be solubilized from tissue by using high salt concentrations or with chaotropic agents,[†] such as 4 M guanidinium chloride, which are believed to exist in tissue as large aggregates. The aggregation properties of proteoglycans have been studied extensively using chondroitin sulfate proteoglycan isolated from cartilage,[6] but it is likely that similar aggregation mechanisms occur in other connective tissues. A few years ago, it was believed that proteoglycan aggregated because of a substance referred to as *glycoprotein link*,[7] which was thought to hold several individual proteoglycans together, forming much larger aggregates. More recently, it has become evident that chondroitin sulfate proteoglycans combine with hyaluronic acid so that if about 0.5 to 1 percent hyaluronic acid is added to a proteoglycan

---

[*]The individual sugars of polysaccharides—glycogen, glycosaminoglycans, and so on—are joined by glycoside bonds.

Sugar molecules can exist in a linear form, but it is much more common that they form a ring structure. To do this, the carbonyl carbon (the carbon of the aldehyde or ketone group, usually #1 or #2) forms a carbon-oxygen-carbon bond with another carbon (usually #5) within the same sugar molecule. This forms a ring with an oxygen atom as a member of the ring. This same carbon (#1 or #2) can then react with a hydroxyl group of another molecule to form another carbon-oxygen-carbon bond. This has the form of an ether but, because it is a carbonyl carbon, there is a higher energy in the bond and it is called a *glycoside bond*. In the case of polysaccharides, the second bond is formed with a hydroxyl of another sugar molecule.

[†]Two molar CaCl$_2$ or three molar MgCl$_2$ will dissociate proteoglycans from surrounding protein. Four molar guanidinium chloride is a much more effective separator than expected from its salt concentration, hence "chaotropic."

solution the two will aggregate into a much larger unit.[8] The portion of the proteoglycan protein core that is virtually devoid of carbohydrate has a high affinity for the decasaccharide unit of hyaluronic acid.[9,10] Although the nature of this noncovalent interaction is completely unknown, there are precedents for such interactions; furthermore, it has been pointed out that lysozyme exhibits an analogous binding to a hexasaccharide in the murein of bacterial cell walls.[11] The aggregates formed between proteoglycan subunits and hyaluronic acid are relatively unstable and can be broken by mild treatment such as ultracentrifugation.[6] If a third component, the glycoprotein link, is added to the hyaluronate-proteoglycan aggregate, a much firmer structure is formed. Two such link molecules have now been identified and found to have molecular weights of 65,000 and 40,000,[12] and it is suggested that the two forms are structurally related and that they act to stabilize the aggregation between proteoglycan and hyaluronate molecules. This "superaggregate" is shown in Figure 2, and, indeed, molecules such as this have been visualized in the electron microscope and excellent photographs have been published.[13]

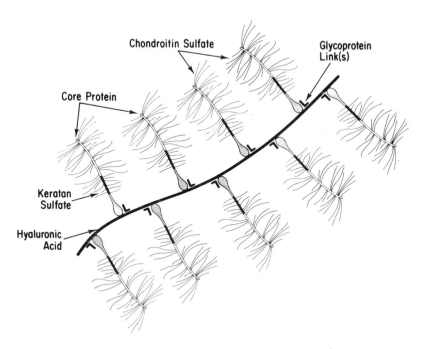

FIG. 2.   The aggregated form of cartilage proteoglycans.

BIOSYNTHESIS

The protein core is formed in the endoplasmic reticulum by well-known protein biosynthesis mechanisms. Glycosyl transferases, which can be isolated from this cellular compartment, then begin to add the linkage region. A specific enzyme attaches xylose to the hydroxyl of a seryl residue in the backbone of the protein core.[14] A second enzyme adds galactose to the xylose, yet a third enzyme attaches the next galactose, and a fourth adds glucuronic acid. This is thought to occur as the protein core is being transported along the lumen of the endoplasmic reticulum. Enzymes that repetitively add galactosamine and glucuronic acid in sequence are found concentrated in the Golgi apparatus, and these enzymes are sometimes referred to as *chondroitin polymerases*. Following formation of the carbohydrate chain, sulfate groups are added to the appropriate hydroxyls as shown in Table 1. The donor for these sulfate groups is phosphoadenosylphosphosulfate, sometimes called *active sulfate*. This biosynthetic mechanism demonstrates well the concept that there is no genetic message for carbohydrate structure, but that specificity of structure is provided for by the presence in the cell of glycosyl transferases capable of recognizing acceptor molecules and transferring the appropriate sugar. After the polymerization of a chondroitin chain, certain of the glucuronic acid residues already incorporated are acted upon by an epimerase which gives rise to L-iduronic acid.[15] This epimerization has been shown to occur in the biosynthesis of dermatan sulfate and possibly heparan sulfate.

Dermatan and heparan sulfates thus contain segments of the chain that have iduronate residues and segments that contain glucuronate. Some of the iduronates are sulfated and, as we shall see later, this variability of structure explains, in part, the pathological storage of these two compounds in the mucopolysaccharidoses.

Once formed, the proteoglycans are secreted from the cell into the extracellular space. It is possible that they remain attached to the surface of the cell for a certain period of time rather than freely diffusing away, and preliminary evidence is available to support this idea. If this is so, then the high negative charge buildup on the surface of proteoglycan-secreting cells would seriously influence transport of other substances across the cell membrane.

TURNOVER

It has been known for several years that, once formed, the proteoglycans have a relatively short half-life, on the order of seven days,[16] although this may seem puzzling in that they are intimately associated in the extracellular space with fibers of collagen, a notoriously long-lived protein. The initial stages of proteoglycan degradation may result from secreted lysosomal cathepsins,* but degradation of the glycosaminoglycans is accomplished in vacuoles inside the cell.[17] Thus, the free chains must be taken up by degradative cells and acted upon by lysosomal carbohydrases specific for each of the possible linkages found in the glycosaminoglycan. Genetic errors in the formation of these carbohydrases give rise to the class of lysosomal storage diseases known as mucopolysaccharidoses, a subject which has been thoroughly reviewed by Neufeld.[18] In these conditions, dermatan sulfate, heparin sulfate, and sometimes keratan sulfate accumulate in cells and are excreted in only partially degraded form in the urine. As pointed out earlier, two of these glycosaminoglycans, dermatan sulfate and heparin sulfate, are known to exhibit subtle variations in structure, e.g., the presence of a few sulfated iduronic acid residues. In order for normal turnover to occur, each of these minor variations requires the presence of an additional degradative enzyme. Thus, in the example just given a specific enzyme capable of removing the sulfate group from iduronic acid must act before α-L-iduronidase can remove the terminal iduronic acid. Such an iduronosulfate sulfatase is missing in Hunter's syndrome and the iduronidase is missing in both Hurler's and Scheie's syndromes.[18] In each, the pathology results from undue accumulation of the glycosaminoglycans. Thus, the more variation in structure, the greater is the possibility for genetic error since more enzymes must be synthesized to degrade the compound. Neufeld has also described a novel mechanism for the degradation of glycosaminoglycans which is apparently obligatory for connective tissue cells.[18] The generally accepted lysosome theory of DeDuve holds that substrate destined for degradation is taken up by a cell and into a pinocytotic vesicle. This vesicle then fuses with a primary lysosome containing the degradative enzymes to form a secondary lysosome. Degradation proceeds and the small molecular weight products are excreted. By contrast, the enzymes responsible for the degradation of glycosaminoglycans appear to be first secreted from the cell, then recognized by specific receptors on the surface of the same or of a different cell, and thereafter taken into the cell, perhaps by pinocytosis. At the same time, substrate is also taken up and these two pinocytotic vesicles then fuse to give rise to the secondary lysosome.

---

*Cathepsins are a series of degradative enzymes found in lysosomes. Cathepsin D seems to be most important and will cleave the protein of the proteoglycan to give a short chain with several attached glycosaminoglycans.

HEALING WOUNDS

Almost nothing is known about the proteoglycans of healing wounds, probably because we are severely limited by the amount of tissue available in an incised wound. The current techniques for studying proteoglycan structure have been developed using large amounts of proteoglycan-rich cartilage and are not easily adapted to other tissues containing much less proteoglycan.

Earlier work in which glycosaminoglycans were isolated from tissue by proteolysis did show that the granulation tissue and even the resultant scar differed in their complement of glycosaminoglycans when compared with the original uninjured tissue. There is not at this time a rational explanation for these observations.

The hypothesis that proteoglycans aid in the assembly of collagen fibrils is often stated. Glycosaminoglycans will interact with soluble collagen. For example, in the presence of dermatan sulfate soluble collagen will form fibrils at 4 C, whereas it would usually remain soluble. Collagen will, however, spontaneously form fibrils at 37 C without the presence of any glycosaminoglycans. Thus, collagen will form a fiber spontaneously in physiologic conditions so that it is unwarranted at this time to conclude that glycosaminoglycans serve, as some have suggested, as a "template" for collagen fiber formation.

Similarly, it has been shown in experiments with "artificial skin" that the addition of glycosaminoglycans will influence the mechanical properties of collagen fibrils that are reconstituted from a solution of helical collagen. The sulfated glycosaminoglycans will protect the reconstituted collagen from bacterial collagenase with maximum effect when the glycosaminoglycans are approximately 16 percent by weight. The sulfated glycosaminoglycans are also associated with increased tensile strength when the percent glycosaminoglycan is increased from 0 percent to 10 percent, but there is a decline in tensile strength at higher concentrations of glycosaminoglycans. Hyaluronic acid does not show either of these effects.[19] It should be emphasized that these are glycosaminoglycans and not native proteoglycans so that, once again, these interesting data cannot be applied to wound healing.

Finally, it has recently been shown that repair collagen is frequently a quite different protein from the original tissue collagen. For example, hyaline cartilage wounds are replaced with fibrocartilage containing Type I collagen, which is a quite different protein than the "normal" Type II collagen of cartilage. Similar changes have been described in dermal scars.[20,21] Wound-healing models may thus provide a tool for investigation of one of the most basic of biological problems, the control of gene expression.

Such a development would prove a most fitting tribute to Dr. Dunphy who, for many years, has stimulated scientists to ask basic questions in the context of clinical medicine. I am indeed honored to be asked to contribute to this festschrift and to be counted one of "his boys."

REFERENCES

1. Jeanloz R: The nomenclature of mucopolysaccharides. Arthritis Rheum 3:323, 1960
2. Heinegård D, Hascall VC: Aggregation of cartilage proteoglycans III. Characteristics of the proteins isolated from trypsin digests of aggregates. J Biol Chem 249:4250, 1974
3. Heinegård D, Axelssohn I: Distribution of keratan sulfate in cartilage proteoglycans. J Biol Chem 252:1971, 1977
4. Lindahl U, Roden L: Carbohydrate-peptide linkages in proteoglycans of animal and plant and bacterial origin. In Gottschalk A (ed): Glycoproteins, Their Composition and Structure, BBA Library, vol. 5A Amsterdam, Elsevier, 1972
5. Hopwood JJ, Robinson HC: The structure and composition of cartilage keratan sulphate. Biochem J 141:517, 1974
6. Muir H, Hardingham TE: Structure of proteoglycans, In Whelen WJ (ed): Biochemistry of Carbohydrates. MTP International Review of Science, Biochemistry Series 1, Vol. 5. Baltimore, University Park Press, 1975
7. Hascall VC, Sajdera SW: Protein polysaccharide complex from bovine nasal cartilage. The function of glycoprotein in the formation of aggregates. J Biol Chem 244:2384, 1969
8. Hardingham TE, Muir H: Hyaluronic acid in cartilage and proteoglycan aggregation. Biochem J 139:565, 1974
9. Hardingham TE, Muir H: Binding of oligosaccharides of hyaluronic acid to proteoglycans. Biochem J 135:905, 1973
10. Hascall VC, Heingård D: Aggregation of cartilage proteoglycans II. Oligosaccharide competitors of the proteoglycan-hyaluronic acid interaction. J Biol Chem 249:4242, 1974
11. Hardingham TE, Ewins RJF, Muir H: Cartilage proteoglycans. Structure and heterogeneity of the protein core and the effects of specific protein modifications on the binding to hyaluronate. Biochem J 157:127, 1976
12. Hascall VC, Heingård D: Aggregation of cartilage proteoglycans I. The role of hyaluronic acid. J Biol Chem 249:4232, 1974
13. Rosenberg L, Hellmann W, Kleinschmidt AD: Electron microscopic studies of proteoglycan aggregates from bovine articular cartilage J Biol Chem 250:1877, 1975
14. Roden L, Schwartz NB: Biosynthesis of connective tissue proteoglycans. In Whelen WJ (ed): Biochemistry of Carbohydrates, MTP International Review of Science, Biochemistry Series I, Vol. 5. Baltimore, University Park Press, 1975
15. Malmström A, Fransson LA, Höök M, Lindahl U: Biosynthesis of dermatan sulfate I. Formation of L-iduronic acid residues J Biol Chem 250:3419, 1975

16. Bentley JP, Wuthrich RC, Van Bueren AM: Lathyrism and mucopolysaccharide metabolism in aorta, skin and cartilage. Atherosclerosis 12:159, 1970
17. Poole AR, Hembry RM, Dingle JT: Cathepsin D in cartilage: the immunohistochemical demonstration of extracellular enzyme in normal and pathological conditions. J Cell Sci 14:139, 1974
18. Neufeld EF: The biochemical basis for mucopolysaccharidoses and micolipidoses. In Steinberg HG, Bearn AG (eds): Progress in Medical Genetics, Vol. 10. New York, Grune & Stratton, 1974
19. Burke JF: personal communication
20. Shuttleworth CA, Forrest L: Pepsin solubilized collagens of guinea pig dermis and dermal scar. Biochem Biophys Acta 365:454, 1974
21. Barnes MJ, Morton MF, Bennett RC, et al: Presence of type III collagen in guinea pig dermal scar. Biochem J 157:263, 1976.

Comment

I have made periodic attempts over many years to learn something about mucopolysaccharides—now called *proteoglycans*. Their structure is still somewhat bewildering to me, and my difficulty in remembering the oft-published details of proteoglycan function and structure, according to Dr. Bentley, is simply the fact that little of this knowledge has ever really been relevant to wound healing. Proteoglycans, however, are both interesting and important. Dr. Bentley gives a lucid description of the structure of the proteoglycans involved with collagen and wound healing and has explained that the relationship between the two in the repair mechanism is still unknown.

I draw considerable comfort in knowing more about the nature of these interesting compounds and having the assuredness of an expert of Dr. Bentley's stature that my failure to understand the relationship between proteoglycans and wound healing is based on the simple fact that the relationship is still obscure.

The Effect of Blood and Oxygen Supply on the Biochemistry of Repair

5

Juha Niinikoski

The metabolic response of tissue to injury places great demand on the mechanisms by which substrates, particularly oxygen, are transported to cells concerned with inflammation and repair.[1] The injury, which incites repair, also injures local circulation. Thus, the nutritional demands of the healing process seem to be greatest when the local circulation is least able to satisfy them. Every surgeon knows that wounds in ischemic tissues heal poorly or not at all, while wounds of highly vascular tissues heal rapidly.

The delivery rates of nutritional substances depend upon their availability, their diffusion constants, capillary permeability, and the distance which the substances must diffuse. The supply of rapidly utilized substances such as oxygen also depends on the rate of consumption, concentration in capillary blood, and capillary blood flow.

The nutritive problems in wounds are exemplified in the dynamics of oxygen in repair tissue. Oxygen gradients are steep between the supplying capillary and the injured tissue a few microns away.[2,3] Thus, vital portions of injured tissues exist in conditions of low oxygen tension, which are probably far from optimal for healing.

Reports from several laboratories have indicated that, in several types of wounds, increased oxygen tensions enhance healing; conversely, reduction in available oxygen inhibits repair. [4-12] A few years ago I showed that the tensile strength of rat wounds increases as ambient oxygen concentrations increase from 18 percent to 70 percent. [7] When 70 percent oxygen was administered, the rate of gain in tensile strength was approximately 35 percent above that of the controls. Systemic hypoxia reduced the healing rate, and the optimal oxygen tension in the breathing gas was passed when the oxygen treatment was extended to pure oxygen and hyperbaric conditions. Parallel observations in subcutaneous cellulose sponge implants containing a large dead space suggested that the beneficial effect of oxygen resulted from (1) augmented accumulation of collagen, (2) slightly enhanced cross-linking of collagen suggested by an increased ratio of insoluble collagen to total collagen, and (3) increased differentiation of wound cells indicated by a steep rise in the RNA/DNA ratio.

CRITICAL Po_2 IN WOUNDS

We have continued the work on oxygen and healing by testing the effects of systemic hypoxia and hyperoxia in wounds of different dimensions (Fig. 1). By using implants of various dimensions, we wished to investigate the effects of dead-space size on wound oxygen metabolism and healing.

In the large implant, granulation tissue grows slowly from the periphery of the implant toward the central dead space, and various parts of the healing sequence proceed simultaneously within the sponge. The outer layer usually contains mature collagen fibers, whereas in more central parts the cellular inflammatory reaction is still progressing. In the thin implant the matrix is only 2.5 mm thick and the tissue ingrowth occurs mainly from two opposite directions. This insures that there is relatively more granulation tissue of the same phase in different parts of the implant.

For studies of tissue gas tensions the implant material was cut into

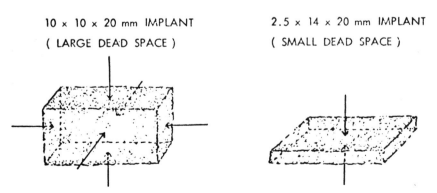

10 × 10 × 20 mm IMPLANT   2.5 × 14 × 20 mm IMPLANT

(LARGE DEAD SPACE)   (SMALL DEAD SPACE)

FIG. 1.   Cellulose sponge implants used for harvesting of granulation tissue.

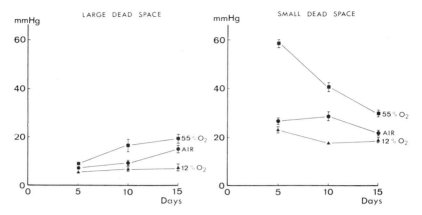

FIG. 2.   *Effect of wound dead-space size and changes in tension of inspired oxygen on the wound PO₂. Each value represents the mean ± the standard error of the mean.*

sheets 70 mm long and the other dimensions were kept unchanged. Tissue gas tensions were measured by means of a Silastic tonometer implanted in the sponge.[13] In large dead-space wounds, oxygen tensions remained constantly below 20 mm Hg under normal conditions and even under moderate hyperoxemia (Fig. 2). In thin implants the PO_2 values clearly exceeded those of large dead-space wounds, and the lowest mean PO_2, 18 mm Hg, was observed on the day 10 in rats breathing 12 percent O_2.

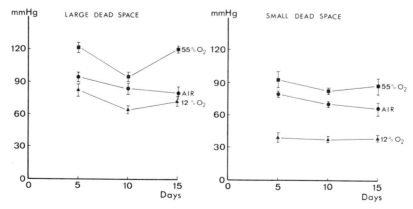

FIG. 3.   *Effect of wound dead-space size and changes in tension of inspired oxygen on the wound PCO₂.*

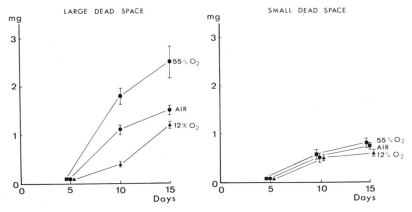

FIG. 4. *Effect of wound dead-space size and changes in tension of inspired oxygen on the amount of wound collagen hydroxyproline.*

Determinations of wound PCO_2 in both groups showed that the higher the ambient oxygen concentration the higher the wound carbon dioxide tension (Fig. 3). In general, increase in the size of the diffusion distance increased the accumulation of CO_2.

In implants with a large dead space, the accumulation of collagen hydroxyproline was almost directly proportional to the tissue PO_2 (Fig. 4). In thin implants, however, the amounts of hydroxyproline in normoxic and hyperoxic rats showed no essential difference, but the 15-day value of the hypoxic group was significantly below the control level. These findings, together with the data of wound PO_2 levels, suggest that *a critical wound oxygen tension below which accumulation of collagen is definitely impaired is approximately 20 mm Hg.*

These data on the critical oxygen tension agree with studies made with ultramicro O_2 electrodes in rabbit ear chambers.[2,3] According to those findings, the minimal intercapillary oxygen tension in the area of newly formed collagen fibers is persistently between 20 and 35 mm Hg. Dividing fibroblasts, which are closer to the distal capillaries, also appear to favor a slightly low oxygen tension, from 30 to 35 mm Hg.

EFFECT OF OXYGEN ON WOUND METABOLISM

Hyperoxia shifts the energy metabolism of rat wounds from anaerobic toward aerobic glycolysis and thereby activates the citric acid cycle.[14] Changes in inspired oxygen are reflected in the concentrations of wound fluid lactate, which decline somewhat in hyperoxemia and in-

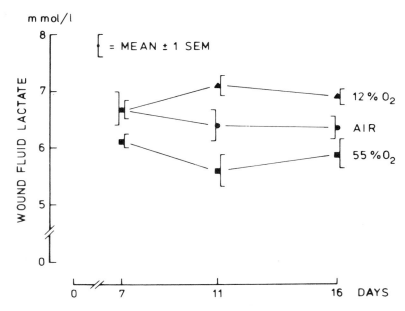

FIG. 5. *Effect of changes in tension of inspired oxygen on wound fluid lactate.* (*Ann Surg 179:889, 1974*)

crease in hypoxemia (Fig. 5). No matter what the arterial PO_2, however, wound lactate remains six to twelve times the blood level.

In hypoxic rats, wound hexokinase activities are slightly decreased (Fig. 6). Increase in the ambient oxygen tensions causes a progressive rise in the activity of pyruvate kinase and a decline in lactate dehydrogenase.

Of the enzymes of the citric acid cycle, isocitrate dehydrogenase and malate dehydrogenase are not affected by changes in wound oxygen supply, but the activity of succinic dehydrogenase is clearly decreased in the hypoxic animals (Fig. 7). The results on wound fluid lactate concentrations and wound enzyme activities were obtained from subcutaneous, cylindrical cellulose sponge implants, 5 cm long and 1 cm in diameter, 17 days after implantation.

Studies in thin sponge implants (see Fig. 1) demonstrate that concentrations of adenosine phosphates in repair tissue increase as healing progresses. The adenosine monophosphate (AMP) concentration was not affected by changes in oxygen supply (Fig. 8). On days 10 and 15 the highest wound adenosine diphosphate (ADP) concentrations were observed in rats breathing 55 percent O_2 and the lowest concentrations in rats breathing 11 percent O_2 (Fig. 9). However, the only statistically significant difference in ADP levels was on the day 15, between nor-

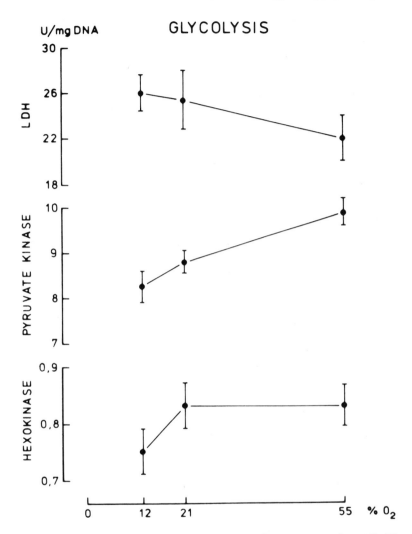

FIG. 6.   *Effect of changes in tension of inspired oxygen on the activities of hexokinase, pyruvate kinase, and lactate dehydrogenase in experimental granulation tissue. (Ann Surg 179:889, 1974)*

moxic and hypoxic wounds. The results of adenosine triphosphate (ATP) determinations are comparable with the changes of ADP (Fig. 10). The highest ATP concentrations were observed in 55 percent O_2 on day 10. In hypoxic animals the final ATP levels remained clearly below those of the controls.

Cellular respiration can be controlled by the substrate level, oxygen

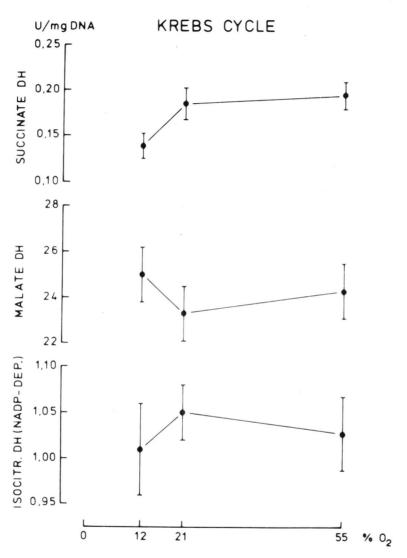

FIG. 7. *Effect of changes in tension of inspired oxygen on the activities of isocitrate dehydrogenase, malate dehydrogenase, and succinate dehydrogenase in experimental granulation tissue. (Ann Surg 179:889, 1974)*

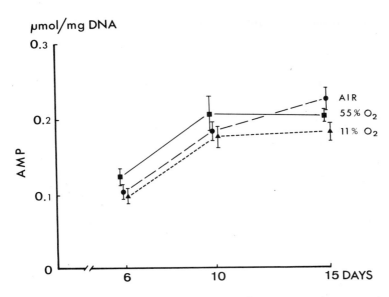

FIG. 8. *Effect of changes in tension of inspired oxygen on the concentration of wound AMP. (Ann Surg 181:823, 1975)*

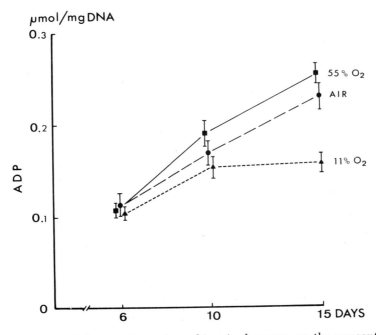

FIG. 9. *Effect of changes in tension of inspired oxygen on the concentration of wound ADP. (Ann Surg 181:823, 1975)*

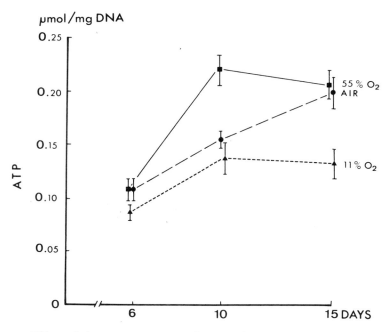

FIG. 10.   *Effect of changes in tension of inspired oxygen on the concentration of wound ATP. (Ann Surg 181:823, 1975)*

supply, ADP concentration, and the capacity of respiratory chain. If oxygen is lacking, energy metabolism uses more carbohydrate substrates, the supply of which may become rate limiting. Oxygen economizes substrate use and, if the supply of oxygen is sufficient, the control of respiratory rate is shifted to ADP or the respiratory chain. The present data suggest that the effect of oxygen on wound energy metabolism is not limited by the amounts of ADP since they increased slightly with increasing PO_2. In the hyperoxic group the high concentration of ATP probably does not result from reduced consumption of chemical energy, but rather corresponds to a new equilibrium at which both energy production and use are elevated. Presumably, the effects of hypoxia are the converse.

SUPPLY OF NUTRITIONAL SUBSTANCES

In addition to oxygen supply, the delivery of nutritional substances at the healing edge may be extremely precarious. It is possible that cells in the immediate vicinity of the distal capillary consume glucose so extensively that the supply to the most peripheral cells is limited. This imbalance could probably be corrected by increasing the mean capillary PO_2 which would decrease the glucose utilization of cells adjacent to capillaries. Relatively more glucose would then be available for the most peripheral cells at hypoxic areas.

We have given local hyperalimentation to wounds by injecting a mixture of glucose, amino acids, electrolytes, and vitamins into the central dead space of cylindrical, hollow cellulose sponge implants in rats. The chemical composition of the solution has been published elsewhere. [15] In the first (the control group) the subcutaneous implants were kept untouched, while the second group was treated daily by withdrawing 1 ml wound fluid from the central dead space and then injecting the fluid back. In the third group, the aspirated wound fluid was replaced with a corresponding volume of sterile nonpyrogenic solution containing glucose, amino acids, electrolytes, and vitamins. Daily application of these nutritional substances resulted .in a statistically significant increase in the accumulation of wound collagen (Fig. 11). Thus, it seems that the wound model containing a large dead space exists in a chronic lack of both oxygen and nutritional substance and, therefore, that the healing process can be stimulated, to a certain extent, by exposure to high oxygen tension or by local hyperalimentation.

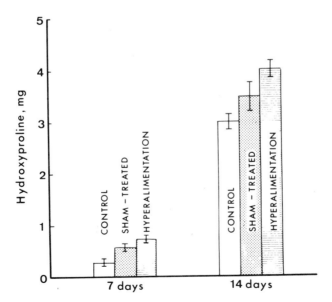

FIG. 11.   Effect of local hyperalimentation on the amount of wound collagen hydroxyproline. (Acta Chir Scand 143: 201, 1977)

OXYGENATION IN VARIOUS TYPES OF WOUNDS

In primarily closed surgical incisions, the oxygen tensions of the various tissue layers normally exceeds the level of 20 mm Hg, which is critical for collagen synthesis. Measurements by means of implanted Silastic tonometers demonstrated that in paramedian incisions of rabbits the subcutaneous tissue PO_2 varies from 23 to 33 mm Hg whereas the muscle PO_2 is between 21 to 33 mm Hg (Fig. 12). This raises a question: Why does elevated oxygenation affect the tensile strength of primarily closed incision wounds [5,7,10] even though they would seem to be above the critical level of PO_2 for collagen synthesis? A possible explanation would be enhanced cross-linking of wound collagen in hyperoxic conditions. This is supported by the finding of Chvapil and his associates [16] who demonstrated that maturation of collagen in chick embryo skin slices increased almost linearly when the oxygen concentration of the incubation gas was elevated from 20 to 95 percent.

Clinically, radical mastectomy wounds serve as a model in which

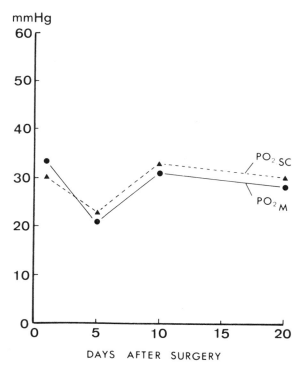

FIG. 12. *Oxygen tensions in various tissue layers of paramedian incisions in rabbits. SC, subcutis; M, muscle.*

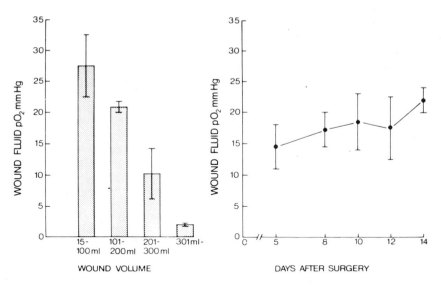

FIG. 13.   Oxygen tensions in wounds after radical mastectomy as measured by aspiration of fluid from the dead space. (Am J Surg 126:53, 1973)

wound fluid accumulates under the wound flaps, creating a central dead space. Determinations of wound fluid PO_2 in patients who have undergone radical mastectomy suggested that a large dead space reduced the availability of oxygen for healing (Fig. 13). In radical mastectomy wounds, increases in the dead space resulted in a shift towards anaerobic glycolysis as reflected by an elevated lactate/pyruvate ratio (Fig. 14). On the other hand, the lactate/pyruvate ratio decreased grad-

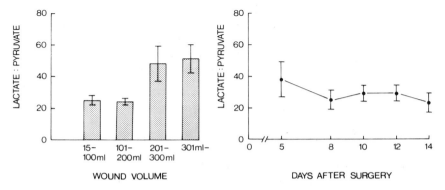

FIG. 14.   Lactate/pyruvate ratios of wounds after radical mastectomy as measured by aspiration of fluid from the dead space. (Am J Surg 126:53, 1973)

ually during the course of healing. In one wound that sloughed, the PO_2 was only 2 mm Hg and the lactate/pyruvate was elevated. Obviously, the most important cause of skin necrosis after radical mastectomy is devascularization of the wound flaps.[17]

EFFECTS OF BLOOD VOLUME AND ANEMIA ON WOUND HEALING

Reduction in blood volume leads to dramatic changes in tissue environment. Fibroblasts in the resting stage appear to be remarkably resistant to severe changes in environment, but those in a proliferative phase are extremely sensitive to such changes. Silver's observations in rabbit ear chambers demonstrated that many vessels in the repair tissue were closed down when blood was withdrawn from the animal. [18] This occurred well before there was any fall in systemic blood pressure; if blood volume was lowered until there was a fall in systemic blood pressure, perfusion of the area ceased almost entirely for long periods at a time. This led to a drastic fall in PO_2, which was most marked at the wound edge where it approached zero. If true hemorrhagic shock was allowed to develop to a nonlethal stage and was then reversed, growth of the wound edge ceased for several days after the insult. Silver's observations confirmed and extended those of Hunt and his co-workers [19] who demonstrated that hypovolemia severely decreases oxygen supply to the wound and delays repair.

In his classic studies, Sandbloom[20] found decreased breaking strength in wounds of rabbits made anemic by bleeding. These animals were often dehydrated and hypovolemic. He also showed that dehydration can decrease wound strength. Sandberg and Zederfeldt [21] repeated these experiments but replaced blood volume with dextran and restored healing towards normal. The study by Heughan and others [22] finally demonstrated that mild or moderate uncomplicated, normovolemic anemia in otherwise healthy individuals does not impair the delivery of oxygen to the wound and is of no consequence to wound healing.

CONCLUSION

Clinically, it would seem reasonable to advocate that enriched oxygen mixtures be given to patients, at the risk of wound hypoxia, since several studies indicate that breathing oxygen elevates wound PO_2 in humans. [23,24] In practice, oxygen breathing can enhance wound oxygenation, but the optimal conditions for tissue nutrition are achieved only if blood volume is maintained, vasoconstriction is minimized, blood supply is adequate, and fluid overloads and tissue edema are avoided.

REFERENCES

1. Hunt TK, Niinikoski J, Zederfeldt B: Role of oxygen in repair processes. Acta Chir Scand 138:109, 1972
2. Niinikoski J, Hunt TK, Dunphy JE: Oxygen supply in healing tissue. Am J Surg 123:247, 1972
3. Silver IA: The measurement of oxygen tension in healing tissue. Prog Resp Res 3:124, 1969
4. Hall AD, Blaisdell FW, Thomas AN, Branfield R, McGinn R, Hare R: Response of ischemic leg ulcers to hyperbaric oxygen. In Brown IW Jr, Cox BG (eds): Proceeding of the Third International Conference on Hyperbaric Medicine. Washington, NAS, NRC, 1966
5. Hunt TK, Pai MP: The effect of ambient oxygen tensions on wound metabolism and collagen synthesis. Surg Gynecol Obstet 135:561, 1972
6. Lundgren CEJ, Zederfeldt B: Influence of low oxygen pressure on wound healing. Acta Chir Scand 135:555, 1969
7. Niinikoski J: Effect of oxygen supply on wound healing and formation of experimental granulation tissue. Acta Physiol Scand [Suppl] 334:1, 1969
8. Penttinen R: Biochemical studies on fracture healing in the rat with special reference to the oxygen supply. Acta Chir Scand [Suppl] 432:1, 1972
9. Silver IA: Wound healing and cellular microenvironment. Final technical report. U.S. Army Contract No. DAJA37-70-2328, 1971
10. Stephens FO, Hunt TK: Effect of changes in inspired oxygen and carbon dioxide tensions on wound tensile strength: An experimental study. Ann Surg 173:515, 1971
11. Utkina OT: Regeneration of the skin epithelium in healing wounds under normal conditions and at reduced barometric pressure. Biol Abstr 45:6289, 1964
12. Winter GD: Epidermal regeneration studied in the domestic pig. In Maibach HI, Rovee DT (eds): Epidermal Wound Healing. Chicago, Year Book, 1972
13. Kivisaari J, Vihersaari T, Renvall S, Niinikoski J: Energy metabolism of experimental wounds at various oxygen environments. Ann Surg 181:823, 1975
14. Vihersaari T, Kivisaari J, Niinikoski J: Effect of changes in inspired oxygen tension on wound metabolism. Ann Surg 179:889, 1974
15. Viljanto J, Raekallio J: Local hyperalimentation of open wounds. Br J Surg 63: 427, 1976
16. Chvapil M, Hurych J, Ehrlichova E: The influence of various oxygen tensions upon proline hydroxylation and the metabolism of collagenous and noncollagenous proteins in skin slices. Z Physiol Chem 349:211, 1968
17. Niinikoski J, Jussila P, Vihersaari T: Radical mastectomy wound as a model for studies of human wound metabolism. Am J Surg 126:53, 1973

18. Silver IA: Local and systemic factors which affect the proliferation of fibroblasts. In Kulonen E, Pikkarainen J (eds): Biology of Fibroblast. London, Academic Press, 1973
19. Hunt TK, Zederfeldt B, Goldstick TK, Conolly WB: Tissue oxygen tensions during controlled hemorrhage. Surg Forum 18:3, 1967
20. Sandbloom JP: The tensile strength of healing wounds. Systemic factors, anemia and dehydration. Acta Chir Scand [Suppl] 89:71, 1944
21. Sandberg N, Zederfeldt B: Influence of acute hemorrhage on wound healing in the rabbit. Acta Chir Scand 118:367, 1960
22. Heughan C, Grislis G, Hunt TK: The effect of anemia on wound healing. Ann Surg 179:163, 1974
23. Kivisaari J, Niinikoski J: Use of Silastic tube and capillary sampling technique in the measurement of tissue PO_2 and PCO_2. Am J Surg 125:623, 1973
24. Niinikoski J, Heughan C, Hunt TK: Oxygen tensions in human wounds. J Surg Res 12:77, 1972

Comment

Perhaps one of the earliest and most definite of all surgical observations is that ischemic wounds heal poorly and frequently become infected. This is one end of a polar set of surgical conditions. At the other end is the fact that well-vascularized tissue always heals well and very rarely will become infected, even when massively contaminated. Injuries of a baby's face rarely become infected. Somehow, in my developing years as a surgeon—and I presume that others have had the same experience—I assumed that there was a point at which blood and oxygen supply became inadequate and below which healing and resistance to infection suffered. Dr. Niinikoski and Dr. Silver (Chapter 2) are giving a potent argument that there is no such point. The rate and quality of repair is directly proportional to the blood and oxygen supply *at all levels.*

Dr. Niinikoski has begun to "dissect" the oxygen effect—a formidable pursuit! He seems to be showing that there are effects on cell replication, collagen synthesis, and collagen cross-linking. There is factual support and good rationale for all of these. Others have suggested that there are effects on neovascularization (Chapter 7) and on leukocyte function (see Chapters 21 and 22).

His observations on local nutrition included both amino acids and glucose. Therefore, the importance of the individual components has not yet been determined. I hope that these observations will be extended in the future. We show at several points in this book that oxygen supply is critical to repair. Obviously, glucose supply is also critical, though hyperglycemia may be detrimental. None of this implies that supplies of one or more amino acids may not be critical as well.

Atherosclerosis and Healing
6

C. Heughan, J. Niinikoski, and Thomas K. Hunt

The concept that atherosclerosis represents a disorder of repair has gained considerable support from the ease and rapidity with which fatty lesions can be induced in the arteries of experimental animals by a combination of injury and a high-fat diet. Despite the many advances in the knowledge of the physiology of the arterial wall, the thought that atherosclerosis is a sequel of injury and repair, modified by the unique ecology of the arterial wall, remains an attractive one.

Atherosclerotic lesions in humans occur at sites of maximum hemodynamic stress. Hypertension is known to be associated with an increase in the severity of atherosclerosis. There are sporadic reports of lesions occurring at the sites of previous physical, hemodynamic, and radiation-induced injury.

Healing in the arterial wall may be compromised for several reasons. First, a major artery is not permitted the luxury of rest—the traditional concomitant of local therapy for any wound. Second, the deposition of esterified cholesterol and of triglycerides may compromise repair. Third, the oxygen economy of the arterial wall may be unfavorable for "normal" healing. Furthermore, any combination of these or other factors may cause the repair process to result in an atherosclerotic plaque.

THE OXYGEN ECONOMY OF THE ARTERIAL WALL

Only the outer two-thirds of the arterial wall is supplied with vasa vasorum. The inner one-third, the site of atherosclerosis, is dependent on diffusion for its supply of oxygen and other nutrients and for its excretion of metabolites.

The outer layer is also supplied with lymphatics and there is some evidence to suggest that outward diffusion, at least of fats, may occur from the inner to the outer zone.

During normal aging, the thickness of the inner third, the avascular layer of the human aorta, increases to around 100 μ, a distance which approaches the theoretical maximum over which oxygen can usefully diffuse through living tissue. In diseased arteries this diffusion distance is markedly increased by the deposition of fats, collagen, and glycosaminoglycans.

There are no reliable data on the oxygen requirements of the normal arterial wall. It is likely to be small, however, since anaerobic glycolysis is the major pathway for carbohydrate metabolism and the Pasteur effect is slight. However, both human fatty streaks, which are generally accepted to be the precursors of atherosclerosis, and the analogous, early experimental atheromatous lesions in animals are highly cellular structures which might be expected to have a high demand for oxygen for cell division, for normal metabolism, possibly for the synthesis of apoproteins and phospholipids necessary for fat transport, and for the synthesis of collagen and glycosaminoglycans.

Evidence from studies of enzyme activities in normal and diseased artery is confusing. There does, however, appear to be increase in the activities of "hypoxic" iso-enzymes of lactic dehydrogenase in atherosclerosis as compared to normal artery.

MEASUREMENT OF OXYGEN TENSION
IN THE ARTERIAL WALL

The technology and performance of oxygen microelectrodes have been described by Silver.[1]

The oxygen cathode measures mean extracellular oxygen concentration in a sphere of tissue whose diameter is six times that of the electrode tip. The oxygen consumption of the electrode is insignificant. Current flow is directly proportional to the extracellular PO_2 and thus reflects the balance between oxygen supply and demand.

In normal granulation tissue, the PO_2 varies between 60 mm Hg, the value which probably represents the mean capillary oxygen tension, and zero. The latter value is often recorded in the central dead space.

In cultures of human fibroblasts, and in subcutaneous wounds of humans, the rate of oxygen consumption decreases when PO_2 falls below 10 to 12 mm Hg. Thus, it would seem possible that cell function deteriorates at an oxygen concentration of around 10 mm Hg.

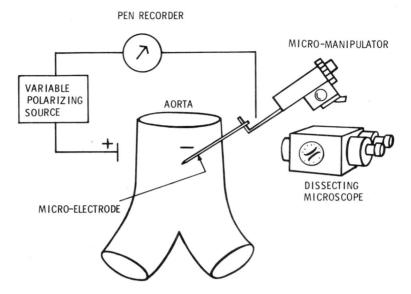

FIG. 1.   *Apparatus for measuring* P_{O_2} *in aortic lesions. The diameter of the tip of the electrode was approximately 1 μ.*

The detailed methods used in measuring aortic P_{O_2} have been described elsewhere.[2] A diagram of the apparatus is shown in Figure 1.

Atheromatous lesions were induced in the aortas of rabbits by preoperative puncture of the aorta with a 25 gauge needle connected to the negative terminal of a 1.5 volt flashlight battery. The animals were then given a high-cholesterol diet. The sites of injury could be identified easily when the aorta was exposed again 2, 5, 7, and 8 weeks after the injury.[3] Measurements of P_{O_2} in the arterial wall were made at these times in the injured areas and in the aortas of normal rabbits.

The electrode was advanced radially with a micromanipulator through the aortic wall. After the lumen was entered, a sharp rise in current flow was recorded, reflecting the mean arterial P_{O_2}. This value was then measured using a standard gas analysis apparatus in order to calibrate the microelectrode.

RESULTS

Figures 2 through 4 show the injured areas two, five, and seven weeks after injury. These hematoxylin and eosin sections demonstrate characteristic fraying of the internal elastic membrane and increasing thick-

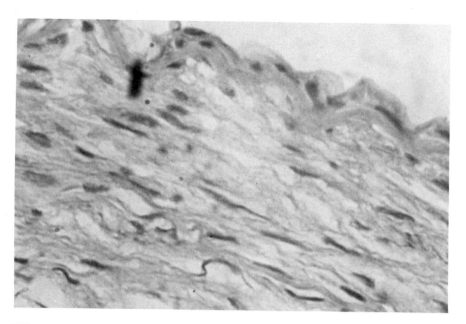

FIG. 2. Aortic lesion at two weeks. Note cellular fibrotic thickening of intima. Fraying of the internal elastic membrane is extreme.

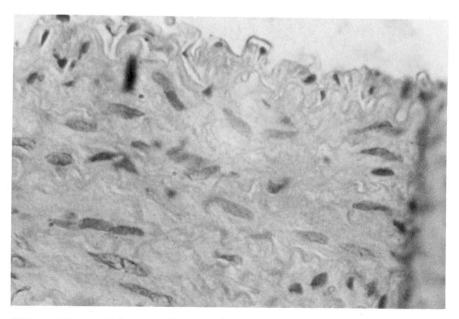

FIG. 3. Five-week lesion with somewhat more mature connective tissue deposition.

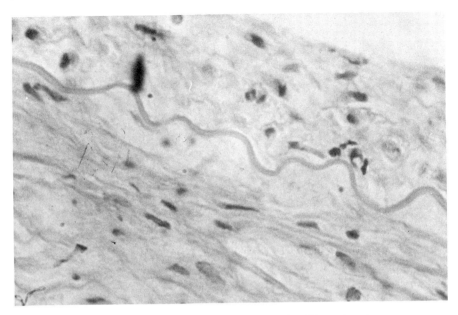

FIG. 4. More mature aortic lesion at seven weeks. There has been some re-constitution of the internal elastic membrane.

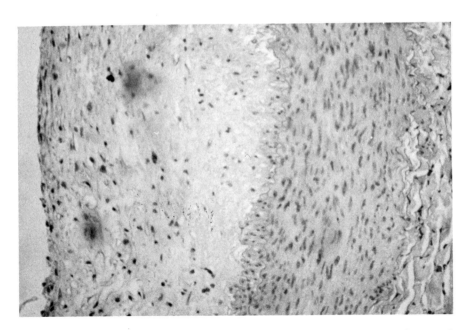

FIG. 5. Low-power view of lesion at twelve weeks showing the thickness of the mature lesion and cholesterol deposition.

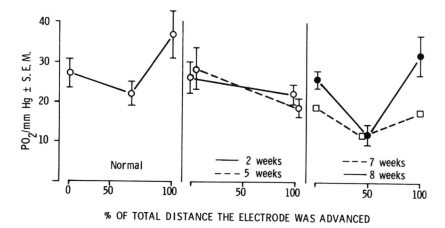

% OF TOTAL DISTANCE THE ELECTRODE WAS ADVANCED

FIG. 6. *Oxygen tension patterns in aortic lesions. The normal adventitial (0 percent of total distance) PO₂ remained relatively constant. The normal diffusion of oxygen from the lumen was obviously decreased at two, five, and seven weeks and seemed to return to normal at eight weeks. This may represent the normal evolution of the intimal lesion since in these experiments no attempt was made to prolong the life of the lesion.*

ness of the intima due to an increased number of cells, together with the deposition of amorphous connective tissue and fat. Figure 5 is a lower-power view taken after 12 weeks and shows an established atheromatous lesion in which large acellular areas containing cholesterol clefts can be seen.

The oxygen tensions recorded in areas such as those illustrated are shown in Figure 6.

In the aortas of normal, uninjured rabbits a steady decline in PO_2 was recorded as the sensing tip of the electrode was advanced towards the lumen of the aorta of the anesthetized animals. After about 100 μ the oxygen tension started to rise slowly until the electrode entered the lumen (see Fig. 6).

The recordings in 2- and 5-week-old developing atheromas show a significant departure from the normal and in almost every recording showed a progressive decline from just over 30 mm Hg in the outer wall to 22 and 18 mm Hg just before the lumen was entered. The value at this point in normal vessels was 36 mm Hg.

Further measurements were made in more developed lesions after 7 and 8 weeks. At both stages, the recordings reverted to the same general shape as in the normal vessels. The lowest mean values, however, were only around 12 mm Hg in both 7- and 8-week-old lesions, compared to 22 mm Hg in normals. The oxygen tension recorded near the lumen in 7-week-old lesions increased only to 17 mm Hg but at 8 weeks had increased to 33 mm Hg, virtually the same value as that obtained in normals.

After recordings were made, the animals were killed, and the aortas were opened to confirm that the electrode had entered an obviously diseased area. After two weeks the injured areas were visible as a 3- to 4-mm white, raised plaque. As the lesions matured, the area of the intima involved progressively increased. After approximately 12 weeks the entire aorta appeared grossly diseased. Representative samples were examined histologically.

DISCUSSION

The pattern of transmural oxygen tensions recorded in normal aortas is consistent with the known structure of the arterial wall. As the vasa vasorum become more attenuated, close to the lumen the PO_2 falls to only 22 mm Hg, then rises to 36 mm Hg, reflecting the inward diffusion of oxygen from the lumen. There is a notable lack of any evidence of significant inward diffusion of oxygen from the outer zone into the avascular area.

In the early cellular lesions, no rise in oxygen tension is recorded on approaching the lumen. It seems unlikely that this is due to any block to the inward diffusion of oxygen. The mean arterial PO_2 in the animals was similar except that at seven weeks it was slightly lower. It seems likely, therefore, that the oxygen which diffused in from the lumen was captured by the increased population of oxygen-hungry cells and, presumably, utilized for metabolism, cell division, connective-tissue synthesis, and, possibly, synthesis of apoprotein and phospholipid. This situation is analogous to the low PO_2 recorded in experimental wounds during the stage of active collagen synthesis. In the 7- and 8-week-old lesions, there was, once more, evidence of inward diffusion. However, the lowest PO_2 recorded in the boundary zone between the vascular and avascular parts of the aorta was only 12 mm Hg. At this level, normal cell function is unlikely to occur and the formation of an inert, avascular, necrotic mass of tissue which may subsequently calcify or become organized by the ingrowth of new capillaries derived from the lumen is imminent.

There has been much speculation on whether atherosclerosis is reversible. If this experimental model is comparable with human disease, it would seem to provide prima facie evidence that, theoretically, reversal can occur in early, active lesions such as the fatty streak of childhood. Later lesions can only organize by neovascularization—a process which may bring in its wake one of the disastrous late complications of a disease whose origins were in youth.

REFERENCES

1. Silver IA: The measurement of oxygen tension in healing tissue. Prog Resp Res 3:124, 1969
2. Niinikoski J, Heughan C, Hunt TK: Oxygen tensions in the aortic wall of normal rabbits. Atherosclerosis 17:353, 1973
3. Heughan C, Niinikoski J, Hunt TK: Oxygen tension in lesions of experimental atherosclerosis of rabbits. Atherosclerosis 17:361, 1973

Comment

Dr. Heughan has examined one aspect of a hypothesis of the development of atherosclerosis most recently developed by Dr. Ross and his co-workers. There are many similarities between arteriosclerosis and wound healing. In addition to the fact that collagen is one of the main ingredients of the arteriosclerotic plaque, neovascularization is often evident, and it is thought that many of the fat-laden cells seen in early lesions are macrophages. Now, Dr. Heughan has reported that local hypoxia, one of the prime features of injury, is also present in developing atheromata.

Earlier in the symposium, Dr. Niinikoski proposed that an oxygen tension of 20 is a critical one for fibroblasts. Certainly, the tensions measured here went below this level.

The idea that wound healing and arteriosclerosis are related is not a new one, and the evidence still mounts in favor of it. With some of the other insights exposed in this symposium the possibilities for control of this major disease seem amplified.

The Healing of Partial-Thickness Skin Injuries

7

Timothy A. Miller

We are accustomed to regarding the burn wound as a single entity. Although areas of second- and third-degree injury are specifically identified, in general they are managed similarly. Because of its greater influence in determining mortality, however, we tend to stress the importance of the third-degree burn wound often at the expense of further damage to tissue which has sustained only a second-degree burn. Considerable information has been accumulating during the past decade about the basic characteristics of the second-degree burn and its response to previously accepted techniques of management and reveals that many traditional methods of treating partial thickness skin injuries cause further wound damage after injury as well as a delay in the optimal healing process.

This chapter deals with the factors that can either favorably or deleteriously influence the process of epithelization and healing of partial thickness skin injuries. Observations are made from clinical and laboratory experiments with donor sites and moderate-depth second-degree burns. The latter injury should not be confused with the "deep dermal" burn which has many gross characteristics of a third-degree burn. The burn investigated here is the classical second-degree injury which is red, moist, extremely painful, and often associated with blister formation.

BURN WOUND HEALING

The Influence of Dehydration

Virtually every current manual on emergency management of burns advises blister debridement on the theory that if the blister and its fluid are not removed, they will serve as a source of potential infection. In clinical practice, however, except for occasional streptococcal infections usually seen in children, wound sepsis arising in the moderate-depth, second-degree burn is extremely rare.

The technique of cadaver allograft has been liberally used as an effective biologic dressing applied to granulating full-thickness wounds before grafting, and less frequently to healing partial-thickness wounds where the allograft was traditionally applied after the tenth postburn day when the crust was separating and the process of epithelial resurfacing had commenced. It was repeatedly observed that such applications definitely hastened epithelization. (In these second-degree burns the blister had been removed in the initial debridement procedures.) Based largely on these observations, cadaver allograft was believed to have a stimulatory effect on epithelization (Brown and McDowell 1942, Zaroff et al. 1966).

Given this experience, it was thought that earlier application of the allograft might achieve even quicker healing, and, in a series of 21 patients with extensive second-degree burns whose blisters had been removed, a *single* application of cadaver allograft favorably influenced healing (Miller et al. 1967). The homograft was applied within the first 36 hours following the injury. The grafts became quite adherent to the wound surface, accompanied by immediate reduction in pain and cessation of fluid loss. Surprisingly, within 48 hours, the grafts became pink, appearing to have become vascularized much like the "take" of any split thickness graft, and biopsies confirmed that they had developed a blood supply. Adjacent areas of the second-degree burn wound, treated in the conventional manner by exposure and not covered by allograft, developed a well-defined crust. The vascularized allografts remained essentially unchanged for between nine and sixteen days after the injury, when they suddenly developed a deep cyanotic hue, became desiccated, and spontaneously separated, leaving a smooth, well-healed wound surface beneath. This transition occurred in approximately 24 hours. Interestingly, the graft separation occurred earlier in areas of superficial second-degree burn, but remained adherent longer in areas that had a deeper level of burn injury. Biopsies of the grafts taken at the time of separation showed marked vascular congestion and intragraft hemorrhage, suggesting that the vascular drainage of the graft had been progressively occluded by the epithelium resurfacing the second-degree burn beneath the allograft. No microscopic evidence of rejection within the allografts was seen. Areas covered by allograft consistently healed more rapidly than those that were left exposed. Moreover, the quality of the healed wound was superior. Areas previously covered could be easily identified because of their conspicuous difference from those that had been exposed. Beneath the allograft, a relatively mature, comparatively pale epithelial surface was seen, whereas in exposed areas, the surface was quite irregular and erythematous.

The microscopic differences revealed in these clinical studies were even more striking (Fig. 1). Biopsies of areas covered by allograft demonstrated a well-developed and comparatively thick layer of stratified squamous epithelium; the dermal-epidermal junction was quite distinct and the maturation sequence was well defined. By contrast, biopsies taken a few millimeters away from areas of the wound which had been exposed showed a thinner epithelial surface with dyskeratosis and acanthosis. The dermal-epidermal junction was poorly defined. Perhaps the most intriguing difference was the presence of considerable subepithelial edema in the superficial one-third of the dermis in wounds that had been exposed and healed beneath a crust. Such edematous areas (which also showed an intense inflammatory reaction) were not seen in the covered, uncrusted wounds.

At the time of this study, the favorable influence on the healing process achieved by early application of allograft was attributed to a combination of three factors: (1) protection of the wound surface from dehydration, (2) provision of an overlying framework which facilitated and directed the process of epithelization, and (3) some form of humoral stimulatory effect from the allograft on epithelization.

To obtain further information, a study was conducted on eight patients with second-degree burns (Miller and White 1972), comparing the immediate application of cadaver allografts with coverage by microporous tape (see Fig. 1). Many similarities were noted between the two methods: portions of the wound covered either by tape or allograft did not form a crust, whereas a crust was formed during the first 72 hours over exposed wounds. Coverage with either tape or allograft immediately stopped fluid loss at the wound surface and reduced pain. Healing was faster in the covered area, and the final result was qualitatively superior when compared with wounds that healed beneath a crust. Virtually identical histological findings were obtained for covered areas of the wound and contrasted conspicuously with areas that had been left exposed (Fig. 2). Although the results were identical, some differences between tape- and allograft-covered wounds were noted. Tape-covered areas appeared to heal sooner (7 days ± 1) compared to allograft-covered areas (9 days ± 1), posing an apparent argument against any humoral stimulatory effect that allograft might have on healing second-degree burns. It is conceivable that the vascularization of allograft somehow may have slightly prolonged separation from the wound surface.

During these studies, examination of the wounds consistently showed that coverage and protection prevented crust formation and

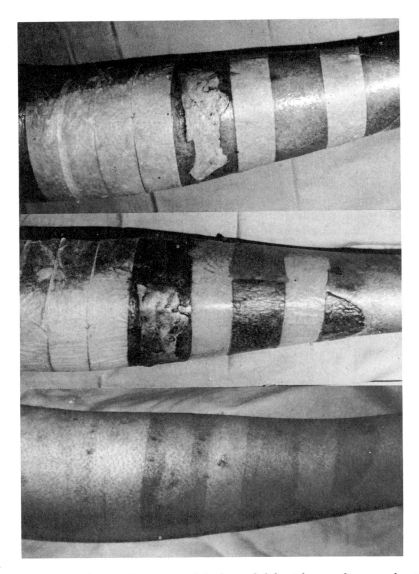

FIG. 1. (**Top**) The anterior aspect of the lower left leg 6 hours after a moderate-depth, second-degree burn. The blister has been debrided and the wound covered with strips of microporous tape and fresh cadaver allograft. Note fluid on exposed burn surface. (**Center**) Seven days postburn. Note thick crust overlying exposed wounds. The allograft is adherent and vascularized. The two lower tape strips have been removed. The underlying epithelial surface is well healed. (**Bottom**) Six weeks postburn. The areas that were previously covered can be easily distinguished from those that had been exposed. (Plast Reconst Surg 49:553, 1972. Copyright © 1972 Williams & Wilkins Co., Baltimore)

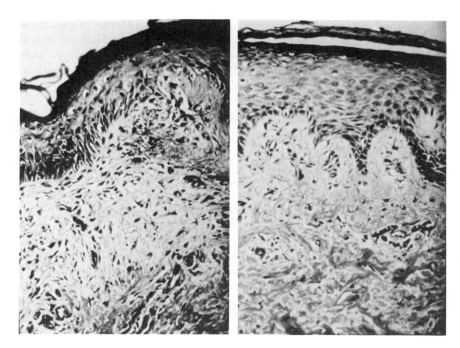

FIG. 2.   Two biopsies taken 2 mm apart, 21 days after injury, of the leg burn seen in Fig. 1. The wound on the right had been covered immediately with microporous tape which was removed 9 days later. The wound on the left had healed beneath the thick crust; complete healing here did not occur until 4 days later than the tape-covered wound, which did not form a crust. Note the thicker, better defined epithelial maturation sequence in the covered wound. The dermal collagen is easily seen contrasting with the area of subepithelial edema in the exposed wound. Very little dermal collagen is seen in this superficial dermal area. (Plast Reconst Surg 49:555, 1972. Copyright © 1972, Williams & Wilkins Co., Baltimore)

that portions of the wound that were covered by a crust always healed at a slower rate. These observations were similar to those recorded by Winter in experimental second-degree burns (1962, 1964, 1965), in which the crust was the result of progressive desiccation of the wound surface and was formed from previously viable tissue.

The Effect of Blister Removal

Over the past 30 years, occasional reports have appeared in the literature indicating that second-degree burns protected by an intact blister heal more rapidly and in a qualitatively superior manner than those in which the blister had been removed. In the management of casualties following Boston's Coconut Grove fire in 1943, Cope observed significantly faster healing in wounds covered by blister epithelium compared to those that were exposed. Gimbel et al. 1957 noted that without the blister the underlying wound "suffered from drought" and the healing process was prolonged.

To investigate the effect of exposure and dehydration on the healing process, a reproducible second-degree burn was created in the guinea pig, a scald injury resulting in a zone of stasis throughout the entire thickness of the skin. Zawacki (1974) had previously shown that if the blister was removed, a full-thickness, third-degree injury occurred. This conversion could be prevented if the blister was replaced by porcine xenograft. In a subsequent study (Wheeler and Miller 1976), it was found that following blister removal, the evaporative water loss at the wound surface increased by as much as 100 times normal loss (Fig. 3). During the subsequent 72 hours, this evaporative loss progressively fell to 20 times normal and a thick crust was formed (Fig. 4). By contrast, when the animal's blister remained intact, the evaporative water loss was normal and the wounds were clinically soft. In this laboratory study also, the most striking differences were observed microscopically. Daily wound biopsies demonstrated that the crust, comprising previously viable dermal tissue, was formed within the first 72 hours (Fig. 5). In fact, *the crust represented further wound damage after initial injury.* Without the normal barrier to evaporative water loss resid-

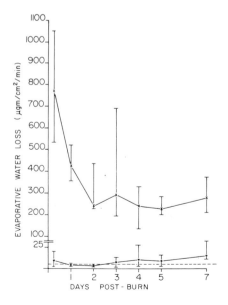

FIG. 3. *Evaporative water loss from second degree wound surface. Broken line indicates values for normal skin. Dots indicate values over wounds in which the blister is intact. Xs indicate those values for blister-removed wounds. Brackets indicate range of recordings, and all values are significant (p < 0.001). The metabolic demands incurred by open wounds in major burn injuries can be substantial if the blister has been removed. (Plast Reconst Surg 57:79, 1976)*

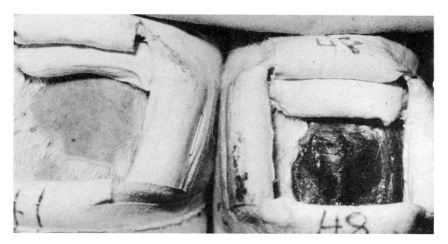

FIG. 4. Five days following dorsal 5 percent burn on guinea pigs. The animal on the left has intact blister epithelium; the wound is soft and pliable. The animal on the right has had the blister removed. Over the subsequent 72 hours, a thick crust formed containing previously viable tissue (see Fig. 5). There was considerably faster healing in the blister-intact group. (Plast Reconst Surg 57:77, 1976)

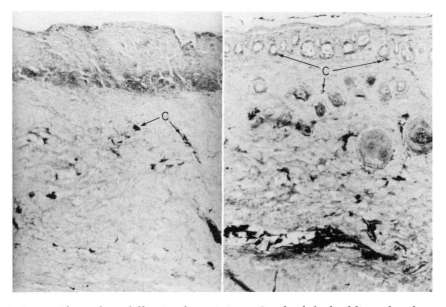

FIG. 5. Three days following burn injury. On the left the blister has been removed; note that the crust is being formed of previously viable dermal tissue. This is not present in the blister-covered wound on the right. In addition, there is a significantly higher level of capillary flow (C, capillaries filled with india ink) in the wound protected by the intact blister. (Plast Reconst Surg 57:76, 1976)

ing in the stratum corneum of the blister, the underlying dermal tissues are destroyed by dehydration. From a teleological standpoint, the crust represents the formation of a partial protective barrier to evaporative water loss. It is, however, a less effective barrier than the intact blister. Moreover, healing was considerably faster and qualitatively superior in the blister-covered wound (Fig. 6). The qualitative difference seen microscopically and its similarity to the histological findings of the previous clinical allograft and tape are significant. Seven days after the burn, the regenerating epithelium was consistently 7 to 15 cells thick beneath the blister protection, but when the epithelial layer was present in the exposed wound it was noticeably thinner. More impressive, however, was the appearance of the dermal tissue. In exposed wounds there was a diminished amount of collagen in the upper one-third of the dermis, where immature vascular connective tissue was somewhat like the edematous subepithelial region seen in clinical biopsies (see Fig. 2).

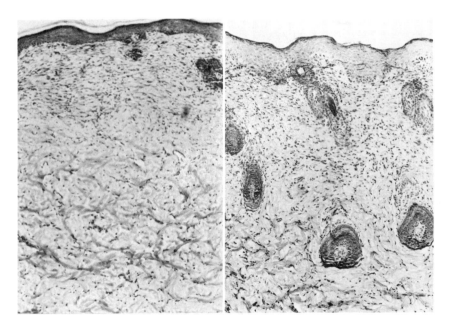

FIG. 6. Fourteen days following second-degree burn. Covered wound is on the right with preservation of hair follicles, thicker epithelium, and well-organized dermal collagen. The healed exposed wound (left) has a much thinner epithelium, and the dermal collagen has been replaced with a less mature vascular connective tissue. Note many of the similarities to Fig. 2.

It is interesting to speculate about the etiology of this superficial dermal edema and the relative absence of collagen. Previous observations of the healing of second-degree burns in wounds treated by exposure following blister removal consistently demonstrated inflammation and edema in the upper levels of the dermis. Hinshaw and Miller (1965) noted the apparent resorption of dermal collagen simultaneously with the process of epithelization. One can hypothesize that the migrating epithelium in a wound covered by a crust encounters significant obstruction not present in wounds covered by intact blister, allograft, or tape. The crust represents not only wound deterioration, but a barrier to epithelization. Undoubtedly, the epithelium must elaborate proteolytic enzymes to separate the nonviable crust from the new wound surface; these enzymes are quite potent and could well diffuse into the upper dermal regions and affect the collagen in this region.

DONOR SITE HEALING

Classically, the partial-thickness donor site has been considered to be an iatrogenic second-degree burn. The fact that this wound results from a uniform, superficial, tangential excision has made it ideal for clinical experimentation. The donor site virtually always heals without complication when covered by a single layer of fine mesh gauze and left exposed. In spite of this fact, every conceivable type of synthetic and biologic dressing has been used—often with less than desirable results—although some of these manipulations in the healing process have served to indicate that there are significant differences between these wounds and second-degree burns.

Donor sites heal essentially by the process of epithelization with minimal participation of connective tissue elements. It is generally agreed that application of some type of covering facilitates the healing process. Following the favorable healing of second-degree burns obtained by the early application of cadaver allograft, it seemed reasonable to assume that similar benefits would be seen with donor sites. Unfortunately, however, clinical trial results were certainly not beneficial (Fig. 7)! Immediately after application, the allografts became adherent to the donor site and within 48 hours became vascularized. They remained unchanged for a period of from 12 to 14 days, at which time focal areas of graft deterioration appeared. As these areas began to expand, they were replaced by granulation tissue and it became quite apparent that a full-thickness wound had been created. Biopsies showed an intense monocellular response and vasculitis which completely destroyed the allografts in a classical rejection reaction.

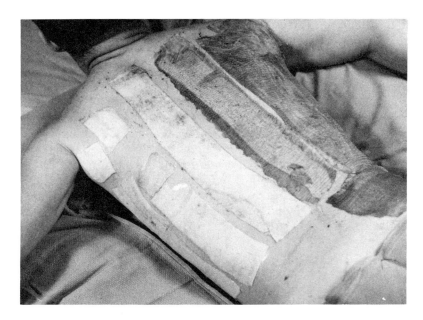

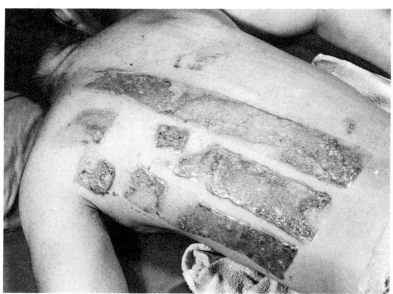

FIG. 7.   (**Top**) Donor sites following removal of split-thickness grafts. Sites on the right side of the patient have been covered by fresh cadaver allograft and on the left side by fine mesh gauze. (**Bottom**) At 18 days, a full thickness wound has been created by the rejection reaction. The area of donor site covered by fine mesh gauze healed uneventfully.

This conspicuous difference in response to early allograft coverage of second-degree burns emphasizes a significant distinction between a partial-thickness burn and donor sites. Although epithelization is greatly facilitated by the apposition of an overlying framework, in order for migration to occur a nonviable plane must exist. The most common clinical example is the epithelial-lined suture tract, where the suture provides the nonviable plane and a directing influence for epithelial migration. Needless to say, epithelium (unless malignant) will not migrate through viable tissue. This is well illustrated by the storage of split-thickness grafts on donor sites (Shepard 1972). After their removal, these grafts can be reapplied to their donor area until they are needed clinically; they can be removed at the bedside with little discomfort up to 10 days later, thus avoiding the use of another anesthetic. Interestingly, epithelial resurfacing of the donor site will not begin until the overlying graft is removed; the presence of this viable tissue prevents epithelial migration.

A similar relationship exists where viable cadaver allograft is applied to a donor site. The graft is quickly vascularized and no plane for migration exists, thus establishing the inevitable rejection reaction. On the other hand, in the second-degree burn, a plane of nonviable heat-damaged tissue allows epithelial migration and wound resurfacing to occur. It is interesting, however, that this nonviable plane is apparently not uniform. In focal areas, vascular union between the burn wound and allograft exist. It seems reasonable to speculate that these areas occur in the region of the rete pegs, which contain vascular tufts that are probably more resistant to heat damage and, hence, that result in a significantly more superficial injury level. The vascular connections between wound and graft occur at these areas and thus would explain the change in graft appearance (cyanotic hue and microscopic congestion) immediately prior to separation. The epithelial migration simply closes off the areas of focal vascular union, and this process occurs before a rejection reaction can take place. There is a basic difference between these two partial-thickness skin wounds; as opposed to the tangentially excised, completely viable uniform surface of the partial-thickness donor site, the second-degree burn has irregular areas of heat-destroyed tissue. The viable tissue in the burn assumes a configuration that may be quite similar to the contour of an egg carton.

The Effect of Donor Site Dressings

The principal characteristics of a dressing that may influence the healing of a donor site are (1) surface, (2) porosity, and (3) chemical components. In tissue culture, epithelization is a random phenomenon much like Brownian movement. The rate of epithelial migration in cell culture can be enhanced considerably, for example, by applying a second microscopic glass slide over one containing epithelial cells in suspension. Obviously, the smooth surface provides a directional component to migratory activity. This principle has recently been applied clinically by covering donor sites with smooth silastic sheets. However, although they provide a smooth surface, they are not porous and do not allow evaporative water loss or cooling of the wound. In these clinical trials, the donor sites became infected.

Similar results were encountered in a clinical study of second-degree burns. Tape dressings of varying porosity and evaporative water loss were applied to the wound surface. Eventual comparison showed that the tape dressings with lower porosity and evaporative loss resulted in infected wounds. When microporous tape (high porosity, relatively high evaporative water loss) was compared to conventional adhesive tape (low porosity), a marked difference in the underlying wound reaction was seen. If covered by a comparatively porous dressing, the wound was dry and smooth and healed normally; if covered by adhesive tape for only 36 hours, the wound surface was moist and purulent (see Fig. 7). It would seem that in the partial-thickness wound dressing, there must be a delicate balance between providing an underlying protective surface, which can direct and facilitate epithelial growth, and assuring an element of porosity. Whether or not some type of chemical component is necessary is debatable.

The traditional donor site covering in use is fine mesh gauze often impregnated with one of various chemical substances which allegedly enhance or stimulate the healing process. For many decades, however, wounds have healed uneventfully and quite satisfactorily when dressed with plain fine mesh gauze containing no chemicals. Indeed, the incidence of infection is extremely low. In a clinical study undertaken of the donor sites of 50 patients (Gemberling et al 1976), each donor site served its own control and was dressed with strips of identical weave gauze impregnated with scarlet red, Xeroform, Vaseline, and Aquaflow. The fifth strip was plain gauze with no chemical additive. The gauze strips were intentionally spaced so that intermediate areas without any covering were present throughout the wound. All wound areas covered by the various gauze strips healed consistently sooner than those areas not covered. However, no statistically significant difference in healing time was seen among the areas covered by the different types of gauze strips. This was the first comparative study dealing with donor site healing in which weave and porosity of the gauze were identical; the only variable was the chemical impregnant. These results strongly suggest that the principal factor influencing the healing is not an antibacterial or hydrating chemical, but rather the mechanical properties of the dressing and its effects on the wound environment. It can be concluded that the ideal dressing at this time is the simplest: plain, fine mesh cotton gauze. Any innovative dressing would have to demonstrate clearly superior influence on healing to be widely accepted.

HYPERBARIC OXYGEN AND REEPITHELIZATION

In the previous discussions, it was appropriate to consider various methods of wound management as efforts to establish the ideal environment in which the process of healing can occur, rather than attempts to stimulate repair above the normal level. Recently, a number of clinical studies have claimed that treatment with oxygen under high pressure (100 percent oxygen at 2 atmospheres for 90 minutes twice daily) speeds the repair process, particularly the reepithelization of burns. Unfortunately, the burn patient represents such a dynamic and complex example of pathophysiology that it is difficult to ascribe any kind of improvement to a single treatment modality. Moreover, the conspicuous lack of reliable clinical controls or laboratory experimental corroboration of these clinical studies has led to considerable controversy and skepticism regarding this method of therapy.

A laboratory study has recently been completed which explores the effect of hyperbaric oxygen (HBO) on the reepithelization of second-degree burns. The experimental model was a scald injury in the guinea pig which resulted in a full-thickness zone of capillary stasis. An experimental group was exposed twice daily to 2 atmospheres of pure oxygen for 90 minutes; a control group was untreated. The presence of epithelization was determined by histological examination following full-thickness wound excisions. The capillary system was evaluated by total body perfusion with India ink. Tritiated thymidine was utilized to assess mitotic activity of epidermal cells via autoradiography.

The rate of epithelization was greatly enhanced by hyperbaric oxygenation with a high degree of statistical reliability ($p < 0.001$). At five days following burn injury, 60 percent of those treated with hyperbaric oxygen had complete epithelial healing, but there was little evidence of epithelization in the control group.

Unexpectedly, upon examining the mitotic activity of the experimental and control groups, no statistically significant difference could be found. The mechanism by which epithelization was enhanced was apparently not stimulation of cell division. However, several other possibilities exist: the first is that HBO may stimulate cell migration. There is, however, a possibly more valid explanation for which some evidence exists in this study. It was noted that in the HBO-treated group there was a significantly faster return of capillary flow to the burn wound. This earlier resolution of capillary stasis may stem from the prevention of initial wound edema. It is well known that one of the early effects of HBO is profound peripheral vasoconstriction. Thus, by reducing edema and rapidly restoring capillary flow, HBO may preserve a larger cell population. If these explanations apply, it would be semantically erroneous to state that oxygen under high pressure *stimulates* the process of epithelization.

HBO has been used in clinical trials; this experience indicates that it may provide a useful mode of therapy in the management of burns. But until more extensive laboratory research can clarify the specific effects of HBO under controlled conditions, it is unlikely that it will be widely accepted.

DISCUSSION

The full-thickness component of the burn wound is significantly more important in influencing patient mortality than is the partial-thickness injury. When calculating the "burn index," for example, second-degree areas are given half the value of third-degree wounds. In a clinical study by the Birmingham Accident Hospital, third-degree wounds were considered four times more significant in determining mortality than comparable areas of second-degree involvement. Even though the average burn injury contains a complete spectrum of skin damage, major attention is usually directed to the completely devitalized component. Generally, the fact that the third-degree wound will not be "brought back to life" is ignored. Furthermore, as long as this culture medium is allowed to remain on the patient, the consequences of some form of burn wound sepsis must be accepted. It is becoming increasingly clear that, although the introduction of topical chemotherapy has improved survival in some groups of patients, topical chemotherapy is but a temporizing measure. The major burn wound is unique in that its dimensions are massive and predominantly horizontal; this fact has made surgical debridement without huge blood loss a formidable technical challenge. At some point in the clinical management, however, the devitalized tissue of the third-degree component of the burn wound must be removed. Without debridement some bacterial, fungal, and viral agents will adapt to the environment and infection will result. Every effort must be made to remove the full-thickness burn wound at the earliest possible time. Whether this is best accomplished by the laser, electrocoagulation methods, or proteolytic enzymes is as yet unclear. This notwithstanding, until an expeditious and safe method of removing the full-thickness burn is established, it is unlikely that any significant alteration in burn mortality will be consistently realized.

With this in mind, current research emphasis should focus on methods of achieving rapid debridement of devitalized tissue and further understanding of the partial-thickness wound in order to maximize the survival of variable epithelial elements remaining after injury.

Second- and third-degree burns are substantially different types of wound. While the exposure method of management is beneficial to the full-thickness wound, it is damaging to the partial-thickness injury. Most emergency manuals currently advocate that blisters should be removed. Nevertheless, on the basis of all available clinical and research experience, this practice should be discontinued. Blister epithelium should be retained unless the fluid beneath it obviously harbors infection. Topical chemotherapy diminishes the bacterial colonization of third-degree areas. Many of these agents, however, have been shown to retard the epithelization of second-degree wounds, and some cause severe pain in second-degree burns. Their use in the management of such wounds can be questioned. Instead, these wounds should be covered by some form of biologic dressing which would prevent further damage from dehydration, facilitate the process of epithelialization, reduce pain, and prevent substantial heat loss from the wound surface. Heat loss from partial-thickness areas often exceeds that of the third-degree component. It is reasonable to assume that the coverage of these wounds by some form of biologic dressing would benefit the general metabolism of a burn patient who has a large component of partial-thickness injury.

ACKNOWLEDGMENT

This research was partially supported by VA Fund # 5733-03.

REFERENCES

Brown JB, McDowell F: Epithelial healing and the transplantation of skin. Ann Surg 115:1166, 1942

Cope O: Management of the Coconut Grove burns at the Massachusetts General Hospital. Ann Surg 117:801, 1943

Gemberling RM, Miller TA, Caffee H, Zawacki BE: Dressing comparison in the healing of donor sites. J Trauma 16:812, 1976

Gimbel NS, Kapetansky DI, Weissman F and Pinkus HK: A study of epithelialization in blistered burns. Arch Surg 74:800, 1957

Hinshaw J, Miller ER: Histology of healing split-thickness, full-thickness autogenous skin grafts and donor sites. Arch Surg 91:658, 1965

Miller TA, White WL: Healing of second degree burns. Plast Reconstr Surg 49:522, 1972

Miller TA, Switzer WE, Foley FD and Moncrief JA: Early homografting of second degree burns. Plast Reconstr Surg 40:117, 1967

Shepard GH: The storage of split-skin grafts on their donor sites. Plast Reconstr Surg 49:115, 1972

Wheeler ES, Miller TA: The blister and the second degree burn in guinea pigs: The effect of exposure. Plast Reconstr Surg 57:74, 1976

Winter GD: Formation of the scab and the rate of epithelialization of superficial wounds in the skin of the young domestic pig. Nature 193:292, 1962.

Winter GD: Movement of epidermal cells over the wound surface. In Montagna W, Billingham RE (eds): Advances in the Biology of Skin, vol. 5. Oxford, Permagon Press, 1964

Winter GD: A note on wound healing under dressings with special reference to perforated-film dressings. J Invest Dermatol 45:299, 1965

Zaroff LI, Mills W Jr, Duckett JW Jr, Switzer WE, Moncrief JA: Multiple uses of viable cutaneous homografts in the burned patient. Surgery 59:368, 1966

Zawacki BE: Reversal of capillary stasis and prevention of necrosis in burns. Ann Surg 180:98, 1974

GENERAL REFERENCES

Artz CP, Moncrief JA: The Treatment of Burns. Philadelphia, Saunders, 1969

Forage AV: The effect of removing the epidermis from burn skin. Lancet 2:690, 1962

Gillman T, Penn J, Bronks D, Roux M: A re-examination of certain aspects of the histogenesis of the healing of cutaneous wounds. Br J Surg 43:141, 1955

Harris DR, Filarski SA Jr, Hector RE: The effect of sialstic sheet dressing on the healing of split-skin graft donor sites. Plast Reconstr Surg 52:189, 1973

Hinshaw J, Miller ER: Histology of healing split-thickness, full-thickness autogenous skin grafts and donor sites. Arch Surg 91:658, 1965

Hinshaw J, Payne F: The restoration and remodeling of the skin after a second degree burn. Surg Gynecol Obstet 117:738, 1963

Miller TA: The deleterious effect of split-skin homograft coverage on split-skin donor sites. Plast Reconstr Surg 53:316, 1974

Wilson JS, Moncrief JA: Vapor pressure of normal and burned skin. Ann Surg 162:130, 1965

Comments

Dr. Miller has demonstrated that profound insights into the nature and healing of wounds can still be made with simple techniques. Using little more than his eyes and a microscope, he has revolutionized my concept of a second-degree burn.

He has made a convincing case for protecting the second-degree burn wound in order to aid its repair, and his suggestions have the advantage of simplicity.

Many investigators have shown that the burn wound increases in depth during the first three days after injury. On the first postburn day, some surface or dermal tissue may survive when transplanted or cultured, whereas a few days later, if allowed to remain in situ, this tissue will not survive if transplanted. It is reassuring to know that such simple methods as those advocated here by Dr. Miller can retard the progression of the burn injury.

It has been difficult for me to accept that skin graft could "take" over second-degree wounds. I still want to know how the vessels bridge the space or how they make a hole in the injured epidermis on their way to communicating with the allograft. His observations, however, leave no doubt that they do.

In his discussion of donor site dressings, Dr. Miller has made a case for simplicity, and he has certainly destroyed a great deal of superstition. To my eye, however, he has not yet proved that epithelization cannot be aided under proper circumstances. I am sure that the search for a better dressing, or a stimulator to epithelial cell division, will continue.

His remarks about oxygen, although careful, precise, and accurate, are sure to be overinterpreted by enthusiasts and ignored by skeptics. One would do well to read this section carefully and refer to the source material. I am convinced that his observations are correct. I tend to disagree somewhat with his speculations on how hyperbaric oxygen aids the epithelization of burns, but I am sure that it does. Medawar showed, years ago, that tissue explants epithelized better in higher-oxygen environments, and Im and Hoopes have shown that new epithelial cells depend primarily on glycolytic metabolism for energy, but will use more oxygen if it becomes available. One hopes that Dr. Miller will soon study the rate of epithelization of partial-thickness skin graft donor sites under hyperbaric oxygen or focus his hyperbaric oxygen treatments to the first few days after the burn to see if the effect on edema is, in fact, the primary effect of the hyperbaric therapy.

As Dr. Miller concludes, it seems highly probable that further research on the burn wounds and its repair may yield startlingly useful data.

REFERENCES

Im MJC, Hoopes JE: Energy metabolism in healing skin wounds. J Surg Res 10:459, 1970
Medawar PB: The behavior of mammalian skin epithelium under strictly anaerobic conditions. Q J Micr Sci 88:27

Hormone Influence on Wound Healing
8

Juhani Ahonen, Hasse Jiborn,
and Bengt Zederfeldt

In general terms, the healing of wounds is a nonspecific process resulting in the formation of connective tissue bridging a tissue defect. The process involves different phases: inflammation, proliferation of vessels and fibroblasts, and maturation of the granulation tissue with chemical and architectural changes of the collagen (Ross and Odland 1969; Ahonen 1968; Forrester et al. 1969). In principle, hormones can alter the healing process in rate or in quality by an influence on each of these phases. With the potency of many hormones to alter both inflammatory reactions and cell metabolism, one should expect the endocrinology of repair to be a vast and fascinating field. Much interest has also been devoted to studies of the effect of different hormones on the healing process, and the number of publications in this field is huge. It is, however, a fact that only a few hormones have significant effects on the healing process in the adult organism. Although hormones involved directly in cell metabolism such as insulin (Rosenthal et al 1962), somatotropin (Koskinen 1963) and anabolic steroids (Loddi and Moggi 1953) in some studies have been claimed to increase the rate of healing, there are also numerous studies that have failed to demonstrate any such influence (Mikkonen et al 1966; Pearce et al 1960; Ehrlich and Hunt 1969). Although the possible influence on new connective-tissue formation of these hormones is of considerable theoretical interest, it seems fair to conclude that none have a significant influence on the healing proccess that is of practical importance.

There are, however, two groups of hormones that have considerable influence on the healing process with consequences in clinical practice, namely, the glucocorticoids and the female sex hormones.

GLUCOCORTICOIDS

It is generally accepted that, in pharmacological doses, glucocorticoids impair both primary and secondary wound healing. Impairment of wound strength by cortisone was first reported by Ragan and co-workers in 1950 and has since been confirmed in numerous clinical studies (Pezzulich and Mannix 1970; Enquist et al. 1974). The incidence of wound complications seems related not only to cortisone treatment, but also to the type of surgery undertaken. For instance, when analyzing 500 kidney transplantations, Lindstrom et al. (1977) did not detect a higher incidence of complications in transplant wounds than in other clean operations, but found a very high complication rate in gastrointestinal surgery performed on transplanted patients. The incidence of glucocorticoid-induced complications seems greater in high-risk and open wounds.

In experimental studies, retardation of wound healing by corticosteroids has constantly been demonstrated, for instance, by measuring wound tensile strength and accumulation of collagen in experimentally induced granulation tissue during the early phase of healing (Sandberg 1964; Ehrlich et al. 1973). The effect seems to be confined to the early period of repair. We have found that both cortisol and methylprednisolone retard collagen accumulation in experimental granulation tissue during the first two weeks of healing, but that the effect disappears during the third week despite continued hormone treatment (Salmela and Ahonen, unpublished results).

The mechanism of corticosteroid action on wound healing is not clear. The general effects of glucocorticoids include breakdown of tissue protein and fat which may lead to atrophy of muscle and skin. Further, glucocorticoids inhibit cellular proliferation in certain tissues and inhibit growth by inhibiting DNA synthesis (Loeb 1976).

Administration of corticosteroids in doses that affect wound healing leads to reduction of body weight. Pair-feeding studies have shown that cortisone administered in anti-inflammatory doses impairs healing more than its anorectic effect can account for (Di Pasquale and Steinetz 1964). Cortisone given to starving rats further reduced the tensile strength of healing wounds (Meadows and Prudden 1953). This means that the effects of large doses of cortisone (such as used for anti-inflammatory and immunosuppressive purposes) cannot be explained solely by the general catabolic effect of the hormone, and that the effects are exaggerated by deficient nutrition.

Glucocorticoids inhibit and modify inflammatory reactions by diminishing exudate formation (Germuth 1956) and by inhibiting accumulation of inflammatory cells at the site of trauma (Boggs et al. 1964).

Sandberg (1964) showed that cortisone in pharmacological doses delays the strength development in healing wounds only when cortisone is given during the inflammatory phase of the healing process. Administration of cortisone later than the third postoperative day does not cause delay of the healing process. We have recently confirmed this finding on experimental granulation tissue using locally applied methylprednisolone (Salmela and Ahonen, unpublished).

The initial inflammatory reaction in wound healing is of importance for subsequent fibroblast activation which results in deposition of collagen. Studies by Leibovich and Ross (1976) have demonstrated that monocytes and macrophages are important both for wound debridement and fibroblast proliferation. Since glucocorticoids are known to diminish the accumulation of macrophages at the site of injury and to reduce their ability to phagocytose (Fauci et al. 1976), it is likely that the effect of these substances is at least partly due to their influence on macrophage functions. Glucocorticoids modify the inflammatory reaction in many other ways that could also be of importance for the retardation of wound healing. There is some evidence that glucocorticoids inhibit the release of proteolytic enzymes from granulocyte lysosomes (Weissman 1967). Cortisone can increase the stability of lysosomes and thus lead to an impairment in the inflammatory response. Ehrlich et al. (1973) have studied this possibility by using "a lysosome labilizer," vitamin A concomitant with cortisone. Using both histological methods and chemical estimation of collagen accumulation in granulation tissue, they found that the delaying effect of prednisolone on wound healing can be partly inhibited if vitamin A (or an anabolic steroid) is administered simultaneously. Michaelis et al. (1974) and Ahonen and Salmela (1977) have confirmed these findings.

Besides having an effect on the initial inflammatory reaction in wound healing, glucocorticoids have a direct effect on fibroblasts. It is well documented that anti-inflammatory steroids have a marked effect on collagen metabolism both in humans and animals (Kivirikko 1970). Further studies on isolated collagen-synthesizing cells have shown that relatively large doses of glucocorticoids reduce collagen synthesis in vitro (Saarni 1977). However, the direct effect of corticosteroids on fibroblasts must be of minor importance since the treatment with these substances, if begun after the inflammatory phase has passed, lacks effect. Epithelization and wound contraction, however, are inhibited by glucocorticoids at any time of the course of healing of an open wound (Ehrlich et al. 1973; Hunt et al. 1969; Stephens et al. 1971a, b). Vitamin A restores epithelization, but does not restore contraction.

In summary, it can be stated that corticosteroids affect healing mainly by modifying the initial inflammatory reaction. This is clinically relevant, especially if other factors which might impair healing—such as infection—are concomitantly at hand.

FEMALE SEX HORMONES

Our interest in the effects of female sex hormones on wound healing originated in the observations of Lindhe and Bjorn (1967) and Hugoson (1970) who observed increased gingival inflammation in pregnant women and in women using hormonal contraceptives. There are also some experimental observations supporting the concept that elevated plasma levels of estrogen and progesterone are associated with disturbances in wound healing (Localio and Chassin 1952).

We have studied wound healing in oophorectomized rats treated with either estrogen (E) or progesterone (P) or a combination of both the hormones (E "plus" P). Hormone doses were adjusted so that plasma levels corresponded to those of the last trimester of rat pregnancy (Edquist and Johansson 1972; Thorneycraft and Stone 1972). Granulation tissue induced by viscose cellulose sponges (Viljanto and Kulonen 1962; Pallin et al. 1975a, b) that developed under E+P treatment showed marked variations from normal pattern. Collagen accumulation was retarded by about 60 percent during the first week. After three weeks, the effect had disappeared despite continued hormone treatment. Thus, combined treatment with estrogen and progesterone initially retards the development of granulation tissue (Pallin et al. 1975a, b). Treatment with either hormone alone causes less marked changes. There is a certain parallelism with the effect of cortisone, although E+P treatment seems to cause more profound initial disturbances than cortisone treatment. Our later studies indicate that these hormones, as well as cortisone, exert their influence by affecting the initial inflammatory reaction and do not directly affect the function of fibroblasts (Hagberg et al. 1978).

CONCLUSION

In conclusion, glucocorticoids and female sex hormones delay repair by modifying the inflammatory reaction. Collagen synthesis, epithelialization, and contraction can all be inhibited. Direct effect on established fibroblast function seems to be only of minor practical importance, but the sum total of effects can cause serious clinical problems.

REFERENCES

Ahonen J: Nucleic acids in experimental granuloma. Acta Physiol Scand [Suppl] 315, 1968

Ahonen J, and Salmela, K: Effeckten av metylprednisolon och vitamin A pa sarlakning. In Abstracts, 38. Kongress. Nordisk Kirurgisk Forening. 1977

Boggs DR, Athens JW, Cartwright GE, Wintrobe MM: The effect of adrenal glucocorticosteroids upon the cellular composition of inflammatory exudates. Am J Pathol 44:763, 1964

Edquist L-E, Johansson EDB: Radioimmunoassay of oestrone and oestradiol in human and bovine peripheral plasma. Acta Endocrinol 71:716, 1972

Ehrlich HP, Hunt TK: The effects of cortisone and anabolic steroids on the tensile strength of healing wounds. Ann Surg 170:203, 1969

Ehrlich HP, Tarver H, Hunt TK: Effect of vitamin A and glucocorticoids upon inflammation and collagen synthesis. Ann Surg 177:222, 1973

Engquist A, Backer OG, Jarnum S: Incidence of postoperative complications in patients subjected to surgery under steroid cover. Acta Chir Scand 140:343, 1974

Fauci AS, Dale DC, Balow JE: Glucocorticosteroid therapy: Mechanisms of action and clinical considerations. Ann Intern Med 84:304, 1976

Forrester JC, Zederfeldt B, Hayes TL, Hunt TK: Mechanical, biochemical and architectural features of repair. In Dunphy JE, Van Winkle W (eds): Repair and Regeneration. New York, McGraw-Hill, 1969

Germuth FG: The role of adrenocortical steroids in infection immunity and hypersensitivity. Pharmacol Rev 8:1, 1956

Hugoson A: Gingival inflammation and female sex hormones, J Periodont Res [Suppl] 5, 1970

Hunt TK, Ehrlich HP, Garcia JA, Dunphy JE: Effect of vitamin A on the inhibitor effect of cortisone on healing of open wounds in animals and man. Ann Surg 170:633, 1969

Kivirikko KI: Urinary excretion of hydroxyproline in health and disease. Int Rev Connect Tissue Res 5:93, 1970

Koskinen EVS: The effect of growth hormone and thyrotropin on human fracture healing. Acta Orthop Scand [Suppl] 62: 1963

Leibovich SJ, Ross R: A macrophage dependent factor that stimulates the proliferation of fibroblasts in vitro. Am J Pathol 84:501, 1976

Lindhe J, Bjorn A-L: Influence of hormonal contraceptives on the gingiva of women. J Periodont Res 2:1 1967

Lindstrom BL, Lindfors O, Eklund B, Ahonen J, Collan R, Kuhlback B, Kock B, Brotherus JV: Surgical complications in 500 kidney transplantations. In Robinson BHB (ed): Dialysis, Transplantation, Nephrology. London, Pitman Medical, 1977

Localio SA, Chassin JL: The effect of pregnancy on the tensile strength of healing laparatomy wounds in rats. Surgery 32:39, 1952

Loddi L, Moggi L: L'azione de propionate de testozterone sul processo di guarigione delle feute chirurgiche sperimentali della cute. Chir Patanina 841, 1953

Loeb JN: Corticosteroids and growth. N Engl J Med 295:547, 1976

Meadows EC, Prudden JF: A study of the influence of adrenal steroids on the strength of healing wounds: Preliminary report. Surgery 33:841, 1953

Michaelis WE, Dietrich RE, Muckle B: The effect of vitamin A on wound healing in corticosteroid treated rats. In Gibson T, van der Meulen JC (eds): Wound Healing. Montreux, Foundation for International Cooperation in the Medical Sciences, 1974

Mikkonen L, Lampiaho K, Kulonen E: Effect of thyroid hormones, somatotrophin, insulin and corticosteroids on synthesis of collagen in granulation tissue both in vivo and in vitro. Acta Endocrinol (kbh) 51:23, 1966

Pallin B, Ahonen J, Rank F, Zederfeldt B: Granulation tissue formation in viscose cellulose sponges of different design: An experimental study in the rat. Acta Chir Scand 141:697, 1975a

Pallin B, Ahonen J, Rank F, Zederfeldt B: Granulation tissue formation in oophorectomized rats treated with female sex hormones. I. A histological study. Acta Chir Scand 141:702, 1975b

DiPasquale G, Steinetz BG: Relationship of food intake to the effect of cortisone acetate on skin wound healing. Proc Soc Exp Biol Med 117:118, 1964

Pearce CW, Foot NC, Jordan GL Jr, Law SW, Wantz GE Jr: The effect and interrelation of testosterone, cortisone, and protein nutrition on wound healing. Surg Gynecol Obstet 111:274, 1960

Pezzulich RA, Mannix H, Jr: Immediate complications of adrenal surgery. Ann Surg 172:125, 1970

Ragan C, Howes EL, Plotz CM, Meyer K, Blunt JW, Lattes R: The effect of ACTH and cortisone on connective tissue. Bull NY Acad Med 26:251, 1950

Rosenthal S, Larner B, diBiase F, Enquist I: Relation of strength to composition in diabetic wounds. Surg Gynecol Obstet 115:251, 1962

Ross R, Odland G: Fine structure observations of human skin wounds and fibrinogenesis. In Dunphy JE, Van Winkle W (eds): Repair and Regeneration. New York, McGraw-Hill, 1969

Saarni H: The effect of certain anti-inflammatory steroids on collagen synthesis in vitro. Biochem Pharmacol 26: 1961, 1977

Sandberg N: Time relationship between administration of cortisone and wound healing in rats. Acta Chir Scand 127:446, 1964

Stephens FO, Dunphy JE, Hunt TK: Effect of delayed administration of corticosteroids on wound contraction. Ann Surg 173:214, 1971a

Stephens FO, Hunt TK, Jawetz E, Sonne M, Dunphy JE: Effect of cortisone and vitamin A on wound infection. Am J Surg 121:569, 1971b

Thorneycraft IH, Stone SC: Radioimmunosassy of serum progesterone in women receiving oral contraceptive steroids. Contraception 5:129, 1972

Viljanto J, Kulonen E: Correlation of tensile strength and chemical composition in experimental granuloma. Acta Pathol Microbiol Scand 56:120, 1962

Weissman G: The role of lysosomes in inflammation and disease. Annu Rev Med 18:97, 1967

Comment

The authors have summarized the current knowledge of the "endocrinology" of wound healing, using "endocrinology" in the classic sense. Our lack of knowledge in this area is apparent, as they point out. For instance, despite all the problems we have with open wounds in diabetic patients, little is known about insulin and repair (see Chapter 9). No one knows even yet why anti-inflammatory steroids inhibit repair, though, as the authors point out, we are in a position to make an intelligent guess.

Perhaps the study of the endocrinology of repair using "endocrinology" in a new sense may finally clear some of the mystery. As Dr. Ross has implied in Chapter 1, and as I have detailed in Chapter 22, there is a kind of "short-circuit" chemical signaling in wounds when the "hormones" travel a few microns from one cell to another instead of circulating through the vascular system. Recent experiences in our laboratory suggest that glucocorticoids prevent macrophages from making or sending the short-path signal. The development of the "new endocrinology" will be one of the major advancements of our time in this field.

The information on estrogen and progesterone may be extremely important. For instance, it seems already that the newly characterized, hypothalmic releasing factors and release-inhibiting factors which govern the release of pituitary hormones may affect our views of repair.

The past of endocrinology of repair has been frustrating, but the future seems fascinating.

Wound Healing and Diabetes
9

William H. Goodson III, Justin Radolf, and Thomas K. Hunt

Complications in wound healing become a major problem for many diabetics. The wound-infection rate in all types of clean surgical incisions of diabetic patients approaches 10 percent.[1] In the special case of kidney transplants, they have a 2.6-fold increase in perinephric infections.[2] Diabetics have a propensity to infection by *Staphylococcus aureas, S. epidermis, E. coli,* and *Candida.*[3] Even after control of infection, diabetic foot ulcers have a protracted course of healing.[4] When it is appreciated that wound infection and failure of wound closure are actually complications of the same process, one must be impressed with the magnitude of the problem of wound healing in the presence of diabetes.

In spite of the incidence of incisions and infections in diabetic patients, there has been very little research directed toward understanding healing in diabetics. This chapter is a review of what research has been done in the field of diabetic wound healing and allied areas.

There are basically two theories to explain wound failure in diabetics. According to the first, poor wound healing is a secondary effect of small-vessel disease. According to the second, poor healing is caused by metabolic problems related to hyperglycemia, insulin deficiency, and/or insulin resistance. The true answer to the problem probaby lies in a combination of these two theories.

EFFECTS OF VASCULAR DISEASE

It is often stated that diabetics have an increased rate of large-vessel atherosclerosis. It is unclear, however, whether this simply reflects higher incidence of other risk factors such as hypertension or obesity.[5] This atherosclerosis tends to develop more in peripheral than in central vessels.[6]

This large-vessel-obstructive disease can be a significant problem and can lead to vascular compromise by the same mechanisms as non-diabetic atherosclerosis. It causes both hypoxia and the "malnourishment" of tissues that should be perfused by these diseased vessels. The basic research, as well as years of clinical observations, allow us no doubt on this point.

Siperstein et al. have been proponents of the concept that small-vessel disease as exemplified by capillary basement-membrane thickening (CBMT) is the major feature of diabetes.[7] This concept is based on studies showing increased capillary basement-membrane thickness in adult diabetics and in the first-degree relatives of adult diabetics, persons who are expected to have a high risk of developing diabetes.

It is probably impossible to know what effect CBMT might have on the flow of oxygen or nutrients to wounds. It has even been suggested that CBMT is the result of increased permeability of the capillary basement membranes.[8] If this is true, then the disease would be associated wih leaky capillaries. Studies done with diffusion through the vessels of diabetic patients are compatible with this theory. Such studies have shown that there is normal, or often increased, clearance of materials that are injected intra-arterially into the forearm[9] or leg muscle mass[10] of diabetic patients. Increased capillary permeability is usually part of the early inflammatory response, but if diabetic capillaries are "leaky" for a prolonged period, this may be harmful. It does, however, seem unlikely that CBMT would cause a functional obstruction of the flow of nutrients to the wound.

Further, CBMT may not be present in the newly regenerating wound tissue. To date, it has only been found in tissues such as muscle, kidney, or gingiva.[11] In fact, CBMT of muscle is found in only 40 percent of juvenile diabetics.[12] The frequency of CBMT increases with the duration of clinical diabetes. This observation seriously challenges the concept that CBMT is the cause of diabetes and suggests rather that CBMT is a secondary effect. That CBMT is an effect of exposure to diabetic *milieu interieur* is further suggested by the observation that normal kidneys transplanted into diabetic recipients develop diabetic vascular changes, whereas kidneys transplanted into normal recipients rarely develop vascular changes similar to CBMT.[13]

Thus, on the basis of present knowledge, CBMT cannot be implicated as the sole cause of poor healing such as that seen in the early phases of diabetic wounds.

EFFECTS OF ABNORMAL METABOLISM

The second theory states that the healing problems of diabetics are related to insulin deficiency, to insulin resistance, or to hyperglycemia. As background, it should be noted that the diabetic population can generally be divided into two groups. The first group are those who are essentially insulin-resistant. This group has elevated fasting plasma insulin levels, decreased insulin output in response to glucose, and decreased insulin receptors; it includes most of the obese and adult-onset diabetic patients. The second group includes those in whom there is a marked insulin deficiency. They often have increased insulin affinity (before insulin therapy),[14] and they are sometimes referred to as "juvenile" diabetics.

The inflammatory response of poorly controlled diabetics is known to be deficient. These patients are particularly prone to staph and other infections as well as to the otherwise unusual disease, mucormycosis.[3] There also appears to be an increased incidence of tuberculosis in poorly controlled diabetics. White cells from these patients have depressed chemotactic responses, phagocytosis, and intracellular killing of ingested bacteria.

Most of the energy in leukocytes is derived from glucose through anaerobic glycolysis.[15] The entry of glucose into leukocytes does not appear to be insulin-dependent. The leukocytes of diabetic patients, however, are known to accumulate glucose-6-phosphate and fructose-6-phosphate, which suggests a block at this point in anaerobic glycolysis.[16] This theory has been given additional support by the observation of Leroux et al. that insulin increases the activity of phosphofructokinase in normal leukocytes.[17] Unfortunately, in his observations, the greater activity of this enzyme was not associated with an increased production of lactate—the end-product of anaerobic glycolysis —leaving open the question of the exact significance of this finding.

In addition to effects of insulin deficiency, it has been shown that hyperglycemia over 200 mg% will inhibit phagocytosis and killing of bacteria by white cells.[15,18] This single finding seems to have real clinical significance.

It has also been shown that white cells from some diabetics are deficient even when not exposed to hyperglycemia.[19] This group of patients raises the question of why these cells are deficient. The answer may be related to insulin receptors.

Insulin binds with approximate first-order kinetics to specific binding sites of hepatocytes, adipocytes, white blood cells, and fibroblasts.[20] This means that the number of insulin-receptor units on a given cell is an approximate function of both the amount of insulin and the number of receptor sites:

$$\frac{[\text{receptor sites}][\text{insulin}]}{[\text{insulin-receptor units}]} = K$$

In most studies, there appear to be two sets of binding sites, those few with high affinity and those more numerous with less affinity. Each has a different K value. Some authors feel that there is only one group of receptors, but that there is inhibition of binding at a given site if adjacent sites are occupied.[21] This point is still open to debate, but it is agreed that the general effect of the law of mass action is applicable in either instance.

One cell readily available for study of insulin receptors in humans is the circulating monocyte—a cell virtually synonomous with the wound macrophage. The number of binding sites per monocyte has been found to be inversely related to the fasting basal insulin level.[22] These studies have found that there is approximately a 50 percent reduction in the number of receptor sites in obese diabetics who have elevated fasting plasma insulin levels. Based on the first-order kinetics described above, this means that there is a proportional decrease in the number of occupied insulin-receptor sites at any given concentration of insulin.

Studies of adipocytes have shown that approximately 3 to 15 percent of receptor sites must be occupied in order to have maximal insulin response.[23,24,25] This is a relatively small fraction, but if insufficiency of receptors is combined with a deficient insulin response, there might be marked metabolic consequences. This is presumed to occur in diabetics. Part of these studies on adipocytes have tested glucose uptake which is not insulin-dependent in white cells. However, the studies on glucose utilization[25] give similar results and could be expected to be comparable to the effects of insulin on the white-cell metabolism of glucose via anaerobic glycolysis, described above.

It seems possible that these mechanisms which have an adverse effect on resistance to infection would also have an adverse effect upon the inflammatory phase of healing.

There is much less known about the fibroblast in diabetes. In studies of the survival of fibroblasts in tissue culture, Goldstein et al. have noted that fibroblasts from diabetic patients will survive many fewer passages than fibroblasts from normal adults matched for age and sex.[26] They interpret this to mean that there is some inherent deficiency in the diabetic cell which limits its reproductive capacity and further state that this is similar to progeria. It has also been reported that diabetic fibroblasts make an abnormal collagen[27] and/or an abnormal amount of collagen.[28] These observations suggest that there may be a genetic defect in the fibroblasts of patients with diabetes mellitus.

Further, fibroblasts have insulin receptors,[29,30] but as with the fat cells and monocytes, the significance of this is not clear. In cultures of connective tissue, physiologic and even pharmacologic concentrations of insulin do not have an effect on collagen synthesis.[31] Similar results are seen in explants of whole tissue.[32] Insulin, however, does cause increased RNA, DNA, and protein synthesis as well as increased glucose uptake by cultured fibroblasts[33,34] It is uncertain what significance this has in terms of physiological doses of insulin *in vivo*. If insulin has a local effect on the fibroblasts in the wound, then some benefit would be expected from topical insulin. A few isolated observations suggest that there may be a local effect, but none has yet been objectively demonstrated.

WOUND-HEALING STUDIES

There have been few studies of overall wound healing in experimental diabetes. They have shown decreased size of granulomata formed in response to cotton,[35] decreased tensile strength of incised wounds,[36,37] and a decreased rate of incorporation of proline into collagen.[38] Studies done on the cellular composition and the rate of accumulation of inflammatory exudates have found that the inflammatory exudate in diabetic animals is deficient in white cells.[39]

We have studied diabetic healing using both incised wounds and the stainless-steel wire-mesh wound cylinder.[40] These studies have been in diabetic animals made insulin-deficient by the use of the drug Streptozotocin. We have confirmed the decreased tensile strength and demonstrated decreased collagen production in the wounds of diabetic animals. We have shown that the wound itself is hyperglycemic in diabetics, although the level of the wound fluid glucose is usually slightly below that of the blood glucose. We have further shown that insulin given in these diabetic rats can restore healing parameters. This conclusively rules out the possibility that capillary basement membrane disease is the cause of deficient healing in these animals. If CBMT were the cause of defective healing, it would not be reversed simply by supplemental insulin.

In an extension of this experiment, we studied the effects of insulin therapy given early as opposed to late in the course of healing.[40,41] We found that a similar amount of insulin given in the first half of a three-week period of healing gave significantly better results than the same amount of insulin given to a similar group of animals in the later phases of healing (Fig. 1). We have interpreted this to mean that the control of diabetes in these animals is much more important in the early phases of healing. It is particularly interesting to note that the animals that were treated with insulin in the early phases of healing (and healed almost normally) were allowed to have poorly controlled diabetes during the later phases of healing—the time during which most of the collagen is formed in this experimental wound model. Thus, the lack of control of diabetes did not appear to have an effect upon the function of fibroblasts in forming collagen in this wound model.

In another experiment we studied the kinetics of labeled insulin placed in wound extracellular fluid.[42] The wound fluid was sampled at hourly intervals and an estimate was made of the amount of intact insulin which remained. We found that the rate of insulin destruction was greater in the 7-day wound (in which the half-life of intact insulin was 80 minutes) than in the 14-day wound (150 minutes) (Fig. 2). The absolute numbers do not have general significance, but the trend to greater insulin breakdown in the early inflammatory phases of healing is quite significant.

In review of our own in vivo experiments and the in vitro work of others, three things are apparent: insulin therapy is much more important in the early wound; insulin breakdown in the wound is much more rapid in the early wound; and diabetic patients have a known defect in the inflammatory response. These observations all point to the early phases of healing as being defective in poorly controlled diabetics. It is inviting, then, to speculate that the major effect of diabetes on healing is the result of a defect in the inflammatory response. This is consistent with the known defects in the inflammaory response of diabetics. It is also consistent with the minimal effects of insulin upon collagen synthesis by confluent fibroblasts in tissue culture and with our own observations that insulin therapy given at the time of wounding (group 3, Fig. 1B) is beneficial even when insulin is discontinued during the later phases of healing, during which collagen is made.

The clinical corollary of this hypothesis is only in its formative stages. We are at the beginning of the process of understanding diabetic healing deficiencies, and we do not yet know how best to manage these patients. On the basis of present knowledge, it does seem that it is important to control diabetes very closely in the operative and the postoperative periods. In some instances, this may best be done using a fixed-rate glucose and insulin infusion and by making other fluid

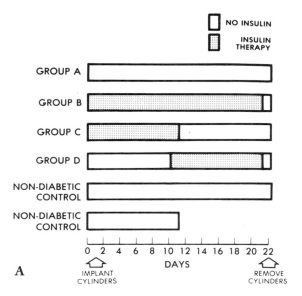

FIG. 1. **A.** *Stainless steel wire mesh wound cylinders were placed subcutaneously in the backs of rats made diabetic with Streptozotocin. The rats were either not treated, or treated by one of the schedules illustrated (days 1–20, days 1–11, or days 10–20). All cylinders were removed on the twenty-first day except those removed on day 10 to show how much of the collagen in the cylinders was made in the second 10 days (approx. 85 percent).* **B.** *Treatment for 21 days restored healing, as did treatment for the first 11 days. Treatment for the first 11 days was much more beneficial than treatment for the last 11 days (p < 0.01) although most of the collagen was made in the last 11 days, a time during which the third group received no insulin and did lose weight.*

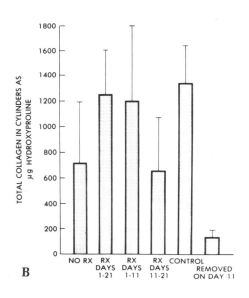

adjustments with glucose-free solutions.[43] Further, since it has been shown that the functions of normal white cells can be severely depressed by hyperglycemia over 200 mg%, we may need to reevaluate our methods of postoperative care which frequently create hyperglycemia in otherwise normal patients by the use of glucose solutions in

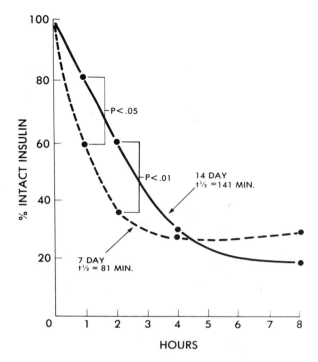

FIG. 2. I^{125}-insulin was injected into wire mesh wound cylinders in Streptozotocin diabetic rats. The cylinders had been implanted either 7 or 14 days previously. After 5 minutes, a sample was drawn and this was used to determine volume of dilution. Further samples were taken at 1, 2, 4, and 8 hours. After a correction for the amount of radioactivity which had diffused from the cylinder, the amount of the radioactivity remaining as intact insulin was determined by chromatography and expressed as percent intact insulin. It is shown that the rate of destruction of intact insulin is much greater in the younger wound.

the 5 to 20 percent range. Obviously, most mildly diabetic patients can still be managed as they have been for years with glucose restriction. We can do much better, however, than we have in more difficult circumstances.

In summary, diabetic healing difficulties reflect a variety of etiologic factors: (1) ischemia caused by large- and small-vessel occlusive disease; (2) decreased inflammatory response caused both by hyperglycemia and by abnormal intermediary metabolism, which can affect subsequent healing as well as infection rate; (3) possible effects of capillary basement-membrane thickening; (4) possible direct effects of insulin deficiency on fibroblasts; and (5) possible genetic defects in diabetic cells.

The adverse effects of ischemia caused by large-vessel disease and increased infection rate caused by defective inflammatory response are easily recognized clinical problems. A full understanding of diabetic healing problems will require further study of these other possible etiologic factors.

ACKNOWLEDGMENT

The authors gratefully acknowledge the review of this chapter by Dr. John Karam.

REFERENCES

1. Cruse PJE, and Foord R: A five-year prospective study of 23,649 surgical wounds. Arch Surg 107:206, 1973
2. Kyrikides GK, Simmons RL, Najarian JS: Wound infections in renal transplant wounds: Pathogenic and prognostic factors. Ann Surg 182:770, 1975
3. Feigin RD, Shearer WT: Opportunistic infections in children. II. In the compromised host. J. Pediatr 87:677, 1975
4. Classen JN, Rolley RT, Carneiro R, Martire JR: Management of foot conditions of the diabetic patient. Am Surg 14:81, 1976
5. Havel RJ: Arteriosclerosis and diabetes. In Kimura SJ, Caygill WM (eds): Vascular Complications of Diabetes Mellitus with Special Emphasis on Microangiopathy of the Eye. Saint Louis: C.V. Mosby, 1967
6. Strandness DE Jr, Priest RE, Gibbons GE: Combined clinical and pathologic study of diabetic and nondiabetic peripheral arterial disease. Diabetes 13:366, 1964
7. Siperstein MD, Unger RH, Madison LL: Studies of muscle capillary basement membranes in normal subjects, diabetic and prediabetic patients. J Clin Invest 47:1973, 1968
8. Williamson JR, Kilo C: Current status of capillary basement-membrane disease in diabetes mellitus. Diabetes 26:65, 1977
9. Tap-Jensen J: Increased capillary permeability to ^{131} iodide and [^{51} Cr] EDTA in the exercising forearm of long-term diabetics. Clin Sci 39:39, 1970
10. Albert JS, Coffman JD, Balodimos MD, Koncz L, Soeldner JS: Capillary permeability and blood flow in skeletal muscle of patients with diabetes mellitus and genetic prediabetes. N Engl J Med 286:454, 1972
11. Listgarten MA, Ricker F Jr, Laster L, Shapiro J, Cohen DW: Vascular basement lamina thickness in the normal and inflamed gingiva of diabetics and non-diabetics. J. Periodontol 45:676, 1974
12. Raskin P, Marks JF, Burns H, Jr, Plumer ME, Siperstein MD: Capillary basement membane width in diabetic children. Am J Med 58:365, 1975
13. Mauer SM, Barbosa J, Vernier RL, Kjellstrand CM, Buselmeier TJ, Simmons RL, Najarian JS, Goetz FC: Development of diabetic vascular lesions in normal kidneys transplanted into patients with diabetes mellitus. N Engl J Med 295:916, 1976

14. Pederson O, Beck-Nielsen H, Heding L, Sorensen NS: Insulin receptors in juvenile diabetics. Diabetologica 13:424, 1977
15. Bagdade JD: Phagocytic and microbicidal function in diabetes mellitus. Acta Endocrinol(Kbh) [Suppl] 205:27, 1976
16. Esmann V: The diabetic leukocyte. Enzyme 13:32, 1972
17. Leroux J-P, Marchand J-C, Hong Tuan Ha R, Cartier P: The influence of insulin on glucose permeability and metabolism of human granulocytes. Eur J Biochem 58:367, 1975
18. Van Oss CJ: Influence of glucose levels on the in vitro phagocytosis of bacteria by human neutrophils. Infect Immun 4:54, 1971
19. Tan JS, Anderson JL, Watanakunakorn C, Phair JP: Nuetrophil dysfunction in diabetes mellitus. J Lab Clin Med 85:26, 1975
20. Bar RS: Insulin receptor status in disease states of man. Arch Intern Med 137:474, 1977
21. Pederson O, Beck-Nielsen H: A study of insulin receptors in human mononuclear leucocytes. Acta Endocrinol(Kbh) 83:556, 1976
22. Olefsky JM, Reaven GM: Insulin binding in diabetes: Relationships with plasma insulin levels and insulin sensitivity. Diabetes 26:680, 1977
23. Olefsky JM: Effect of dexamethasone on insulin binding, glucose transport, and glucose oxidation of isolated rat adipocytes. J Clin Invest 56:1499, 1975
24. Olefsky JM, Jen P, Reaven GM: Insulin binding to isolated adipocytes. Diabetes 23:565, 1974
25. Kono T, Barham FW: The relationship between the insulin-binding capacity of fat cells and the cellular response to insulin: Studies with intact and trypsin-treated fat cells. J Biol Chem 246:6210, 1971
26. Goldstein S, Niewiarowski S, Singal DP: Pathological implications of cell aging in vitro. Fed Proc 34:56, 1975
27. Kohn RR, Mensse S: Abnormal collagen in cultures of fibroblasts from human beings with diabetes mellitus. Biochem Biophys Res Comm 76:765, 1977
28. Rowe DW, Starman BJ, Fujimoto WY, Williams RH: Abnormalities in proliferation and protein synthesis in skin fibroblast cultures from patients with diabetes mellitus. Diabetes 26:284, 1977
29. Gavin JR III, Roth J, Jen P, Freychet P: Insulin receptors in human circulating cells and fibroblasts. Proc Nat Acad Sci USA 69:747, 1972
30. Rechler MM, Podskalny JM: Insulin receptors in cultured human fibroblasts. Diabetes 25:250, 1976
31. Villee DB, Powers ML: Effect of glucose and insulin on collagen secretion by human skin fibroblasts in vitro. Nature 268:156, 1977.
32. Perlish JS, Bashey RI, Fleischmajer R: The in vitro effect of insulin on collagen synthesis in embryonic chick tibia (37196). Proc Soc Exp Biol Med 142:1152, 1973
33. Fujimoto WY, Williams RH: Insulin action on the cultured human fibroblast: Glucose uptake, protein synthesis, RNA synthesis. Diabetes 23:443, 1974
34. Baseman JB, Paolini D Jr, Amos H: Stimulation by insulin of RNA synthesis in chick fibroblasts. J Cell Biol 60:54, 1974
35. Nagy S, Redei A, Karadi S: Studies on granulation tissue production in alloxan-diabetic rats. J Endocrinol 22:143, 1961
36. Rosenthal S, Lerner B, DiBiase F, Enquist IF: Relation of strength to composition in diabetic wounds. Surg Gynecol Obstet 115:437, 1962

37. Prakash K, Pundit P, Sharma KL: Studies in wound healing in experimental diabetes. Int Surg 59:25, 1974
38. Arquilla ER, Weringer EJ, Nakajo M: Wound healing: A model for the study of diabetic angiopathy. Diabetes 13 (Suppl 2):811, 1977
39. Perillie PE, Nolan JP, Finch SC: Studies of the resistance to infection in diabetes mellitus: Local exudative cellular response. J Lab Clin Med 59:1008, 1962
40. Goodson WH III, Hunt TK: Studies of wound healing in experimental diabetes mellitus. J Surg Res 22:221, 1977
41. Goodson WH III, Hunt TK: Wound healing in experimental diabetes: The importance of early insulin therapy, in preparation
42. Radolf JD, Hunt TK: Unpublished data
43. Meyer EJ, Lorenzi M, Bohannan NV, Amend W, Feduska NJ, Salvatierra O, Forsham PH: Diabetic management by insulin infusion during major surgery. Am J Surg 137:323, 1979

Comment

Over the last 50 years, the outlook for diabetics undergoing surgery has markedly improved. In a collective review in 1902, Phillips reported 12 percent mortality from wound complications alone in a series of 90 clean operations in diabetics. Another 12 percent died of diabetic coma.

By 1920, it was understood that diet alone would control many diabetics and results of surgery improved. That year, the Mayo Clinic reported survival in 95 percent of their diabetic patients undergoing surgery.

With the availability of insulin in 1924, possibilities expanded to include surgery in acutely ill or infected patients. By 1940, Green reported comparable results of surgery in diabetics and nondiabetics at the University of Iowa. This improvement occurred before antibiotics became generally available.

The change that occurred in this 40-year period from 1900 to 1940 was that we learned how to control diabetes. Results of surgery improved in parallel. We learned very little, however, about how control affects healing in diabetes, and that defect in our knowledge now seems important.

Other investigators have shown that acute insulin deficiency will adversely affect healing. Dr. Goodson has begun to dissect the effects of insulin (and its deficiency) on healing. His initial studies clearly have shown a greater need for insulin in the early phases of healing and a relative lack of need in the later phases. This parallels the widely known clinical observation that diabetics have defects in their inflammatory response. This defective healing in diabetes may be another manifestation of defective white-cell function.

Collagen Morphology in Normal and Wound Tissue

10

J. C. Forrester

Wound healing is, at its best, imperfect, yet most wounds heal un-eventfully and are soon forgotten. In practice, therefore, quality control is best directed at those wounds that may fail to reach nature's stand-ard, rather than attempting to produce supernormal healing.

Impairment or abnormality in healing usually presents as *dehis-cence, pathological fibrosis,* or *infection.* Dehiscence results when strength is impaired.[1] Fibrosis is an abnormal "overhealing" state.[2] Infection increases the likelihood of dehiscence by delaying strength recovery and softening the wound edges.[3]

The wound is a fiber-gel composite,[4,5,6] but its components can be usefully studied individually. Recent work on wound collagen mor-phology helps explain both dehiscence and fibrosis.

WOUND STRENGTH

Wound strength develops slowly.[7] The ability to resist rupture is de-termined by tensile strength and pliability (extensibility).[8,9] By them-selves, these measures provide limited information, but taken together they express real wound strength, or the amount of energy that the wound will absorb before it breaks (Fig. 1). Bioengineering studies show that the apparently well-healed wound is remarkably weak.[8,9] At 10 days, it has very little strength, but thereafter it picks up quite rapidly until by three months it is half as strong as normal tissue. The further passage of time has little effect, and the scar appears to be

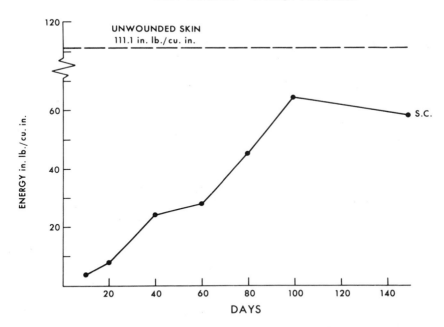

SKIN WOUNDS   ENERGY ABSORBED

FIG. 1.   The ability of a wound to resist rupture expressed as its energy absorption. There is only a 60 percent recovery by 150 days. (Reproduced by permission from JC Forrester et al: J Surg Res 9:207, 1969)

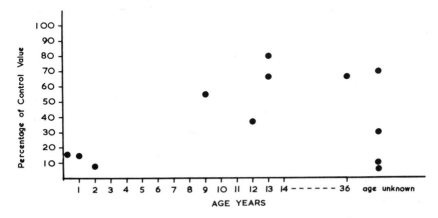

FIG. 2.   The tensile strength of human skin wounds expressed as a percentage of that of intact skin. In the first two-year period, skin wounds are less than 20 percent of control value, and even at 13 years, there is still quite a marked weakness. (Reproduced by permission from DM Douglas et al: Br J Surg 56:219, 1969)

permanently weak. Human wounds (Fig. 2) show the same general pattern with maximal recovery of only about 75 percent even after 36 years. Many wounds are a good deal weaker.[10]

The strength of connective tissue repair is determined by the fibrous protein collagen.[11-14] The histological features of scar collagen are distinctly different from those of unwounded tissues. The most obvious difference is in collagen-bundle size.[10] At 40 days, there is still a striking physical difference (Fig. 3). Wound collagen bundles are a good deal narrower than normal. Polarized-light studies show that there is, in addition, a more generalized disorganization of the wound collagen

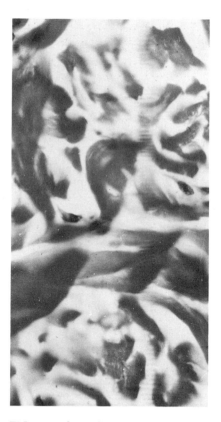 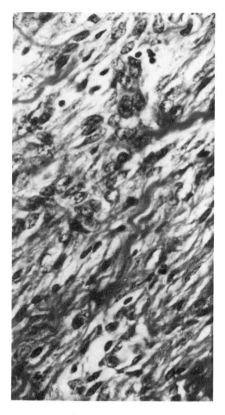

FIG. 3. The collagen bundles in a healing wound (right) and normal guinea pig skin (left). Note the fine-character bundles of wound collagen compared with the large bundles of normal dermal collagen (×250). (Reproduced by permission from DM Douglas et al: Br J Surg 56:219, 1969)

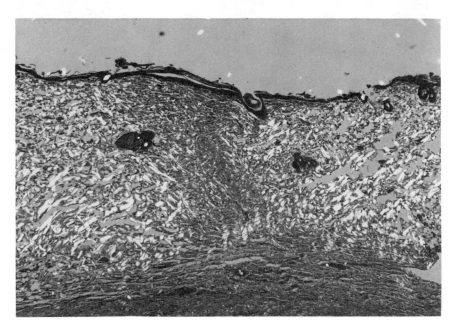

FIG. 4. *Photomicrograph of 100-day wound viewed in polarized light. The normal dermal collagen on either side of the wound indicates a failure of organization of the collagen fiber subunits normally birefringent in the wound (light microscope, ×45). From Dunphy JE, Van Winkle W (eds): Repair and Regeneration, p 77. Copyright © 1969 McGraw-Hill. Used with permission of McGraw-Hill Book Co.*

(Fig. 4). Normal collagen is birefringent; but even after 100 days, wound collagen stands out clearly as nonbirefringent material. This lack of birefringence indicates a relatively disorganized structure at the molecular or small-fibril level.[15,16]

Physical irregularities in fiber shape and "weave" are more readily appreciated by scanning electron microscope examination.[17] At low magnification, the interlacing collagen fiber pattern of normal skin is clear (Fig. 5); this magnification is equivalent to that of the oil-immersion light-microscope image. At higher magnification, the individual collagen fibers are clear (Fig. 6). At still higher magnification, cross-banding of individual collagen fibers is sometimes seen (Fig. 7). The healing wound presents a very different pattern. At ten days, the fibers lie in relatively haphazard fashion (Figs. 8 and 9). As time goes by, the randomly dispersed collagen fibrils coalesce to form irregular masses

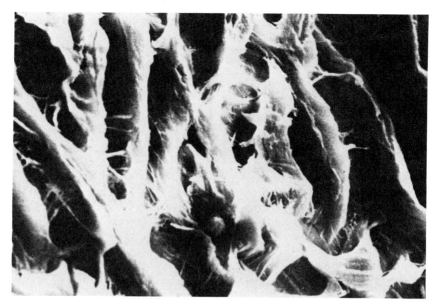

FIG. 5. Scanning electron micrograph of a section of normal skin showing part of the interlacing network of collagen fibers (× 850). (Reproduced by permission from JC Forrester et al: Nature 221:373, 1969)

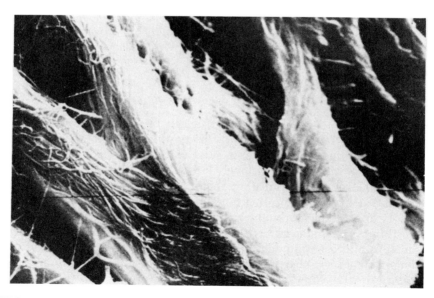

FIG. 6. Collagen fiber network of unwounded skin; fibril substructure (scanning electron microscope ×4000). From Dunphy JE, Van Winkle W (eds): Repair and Regeneration, p 78. Copyright © 1969 McGraw-Hill. Used with permission of McGraw-Hill Book Co.

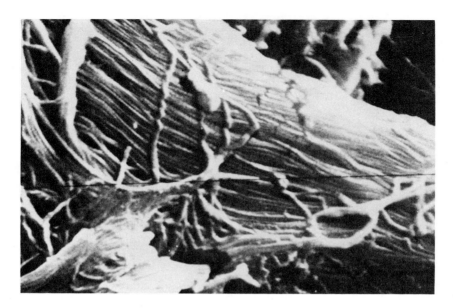

FIG. 7. Scanning electron micrograph of part of a normal collagen fiber showing that it is made up of bundles of cross-banded fibrils (×13,000). (Reproduced by permission from JC Forrester et al: Nature, 221:373, 1969)

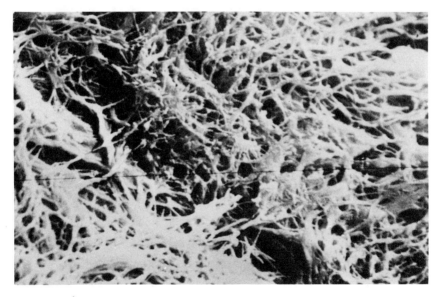

FIG. 8. Scanning electron micrograph of a representative portion of a 10-day-old sutured wound (×4000). The fibrils lie haphazardly. Compare with the unwounded skin shown in Figure 6 at the same magnification. From JC Forrester et al: J Trauma 10:770, 1970. Copyright © 1970 Williams and Wilkins Co., Baltimore)

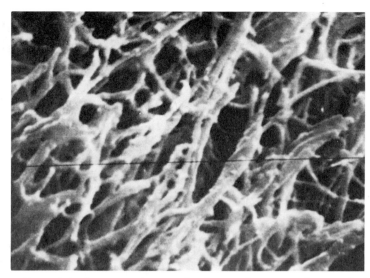

FIG. 9. Scanning electron micrograph of a 10-day sutured wound showing the randomly oriented collagen fibrils. They show little tendency to aggregate. Cross-banding is not apparent. Compare with the normal skin shown in Figure 7 at the same magnification (×13,000). (Reproduced by permission from JC Forrester et al: Nature, 221:373, 1969)

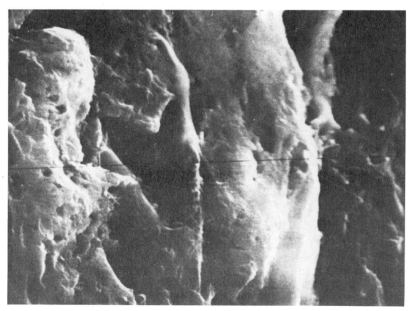

FIG. 10. Scanning electron micrograph of a representative portion of a 100-day wound. The collagen fibrils have aggregated to form large collagen masses, but the normal network architecture has not been restored (×4000). Compare with the unwounded skin in Figure 6.

of collagen (Fig. 10). The overall pattern, however, is far from normal, and close examination of any one area shows no evidence of collagen fibril substructure. The microarchitecture of the wound is distinctly abnormal, and there is little or no evidence of remodeling, even at much later periods of time.

These persisting structural abnormalities help explain why the wound remains weak and brittle for so long. The importance of collagen fiber patterns can be demonstrated by a simple experiment. When tape-closed and sutured skin wounds are both allowed to heal synchronously in the same animal, they show marked differences in degree of tensile-strength recovery.[15,18,19] After 60 days, the tape-closed wound recovers almost 90 percent of the tensile strength of normal tissues, whereas the sutured wound makes only a 70 percent recovery (Fig. 11). Light microscopy reveals that the sutured wound heals in a linear fashion because the subcutaneous muscle does not retract (Fig. 12). In the tape-closed wound, there is progressive retraction of the cut edges of the subcutaneous muscle. The resulting wound scar adopts a triangular shape (Fig. 13), and scanning microscope examination shows a distinct orientation of the new collagen fibers across the wound (Fig. 14).[19] This small-fiber orientation could explain the increased tensile strength found in the tape-closed wound. Such orientation should be accompanied by a loss of pliability, since this is normally accounted for by a flexible network organization such as is

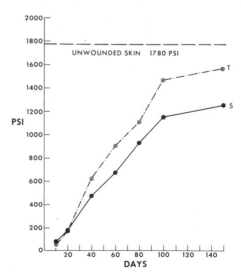

FIG. 11. *Mean tensile strength of tape-closed (T) and sutured (S) wounds in rat skin in pounds per square inch. Both gain strength with time but the tape-closed significantly more than the sutured. By 150 days, it has recovered 90 percent of the strength of unwounded skin, whereas the sutured one has regained only 70 percent. From Dunphy JE, Van Winkle W (eds): Repair and Regeneration, p 75. Copyright © 1969 McGraw-Hill. Used with permission of McGraw-Hill Book Co.*

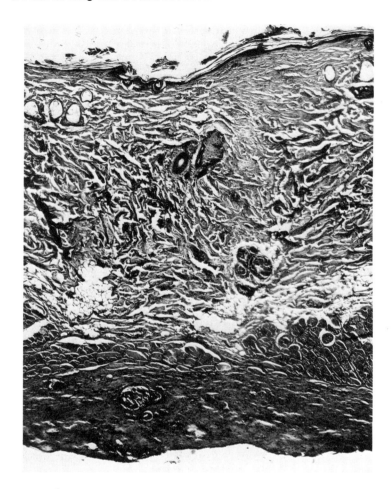

FIG. 12.   Light microscope view of suture-closed wound (100 days). The wound cleft is linear and collagen fibers are irregularly arranged. The subcutaneous muscle has not retracted (×50). (Reproduced by permission from JC Forrester et al: Br J Surg 57:729, 1970)

readily observed in normal skin. Mechanical studies confirm this. The tape-closed wound is more brittle than the sutured wound. This offsets the higher tensile strength of the taped wound, and the end result is that both wound types have the same ability to resist rupture (Fig. 15).[19] In clinical terms, there is nothing to choose between them in terms of mechanical properties.

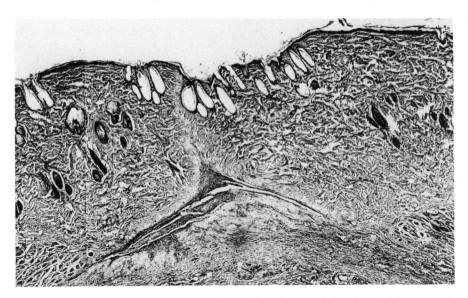

FIG. 13.   Light microscope view of tape-closed wound (10 days). The wound cleft is broad owing to retraction of the subcutaneous muscle. The collagen fibers are aligned across the wound (×18). (Reproduced by permission from JC Forrester et al: Br J Surg 57:729, 1970).

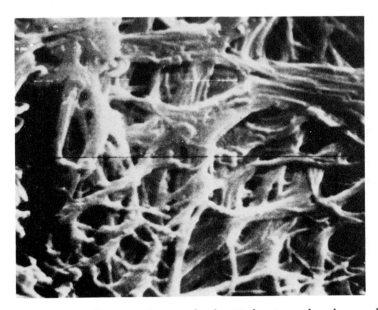

FIG. 14.   Scanning electron micrograph of a 10-day tape-closed wound. The fibrils are aggregating to form small bundles and tend to be oriented across the wound. There is no evidence of cross-banding (×13,000). Compare with the sutured wound shown in Figure 9 at the same magnification. (Reproduced by permission from JC Forrester et al: Br J Surg 57:729, 1970)

127

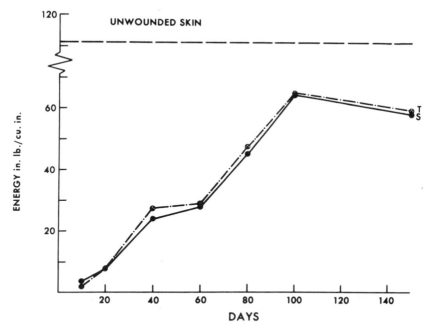

FIG. 15.   Mean values of energy absorption of tape-closed (T) and sutured (S) wounds, expressed in inch-pounds per cubic inch of tissue tested. There is no significant difference between the wounds and only a 60 percent recovery of the unwounded value by 150 days. (Reproduced by permission from JC Forrester et al: Br J Surg 57:729, 1970)

WOUND FIBROSIS

Connective tissue formation is not confined to healing knife wounds. It follows in the wake of many types of tissue injury due to disease processes. Where elasticity and movement are important qualities, scar tissue causes problems. Apart from its intrinsically weak and brittle nature, scar has an unfortunate tendency to contract abnormally, causing late effects often more serious than the original injury.[2,20,21] Familiar examples include the stenosing mitral valve following years after a bout of acute rheumatic valvulitis, the benign esophageal stricture following in the wake of repeated attacks of acute esophagitis, peritoneal adhesions, and the posttraumatic cerebral scar. A considerable number of human afflictions would be alleviated if this fibrosis could be controlled. There is evidence that the abnormal collagen-fiber patterns in the scar are responsible for many of these unfortunate results. If the fiber pattern could be improved, contraction and weakness might be avoided. Physical methods such as the tape-closure technique shown above appear to be of limited value, but chemical treatments hold considerable promise.[12,20–23] Newly deposited collagen lies haphazardly in the wound. Unfortunately, it appears to be fixed irretrievably in this pattern by rapid intermolecular cross-linking.[5,12,24] If the cross-linking could be delayed, then in theory the collagen molecules would be free to reorganize into more useful and more physiological patterns.

Collagen is so widespread in the body that it would appear to be impossible to interfere with its cross-linking without seriously affecting the general health of the individual. Recent studies in wound collagen metabolism show, however, that the wound has a considerably higher turnover rate than the rest of the body (Fig. 16).[2,25,26,27] This makes it particularly susceptible to chemical treatments.

There are three ways in which wound collagen might be manipulated.[2,22]

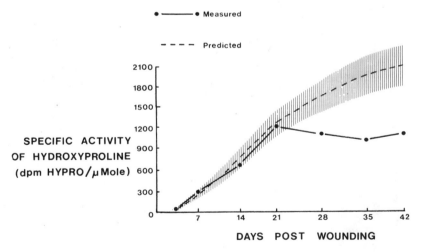

FIG. 16. *Comparison of scar collagen accumulation predicted from its rate of synthesis with that actually measured. Total collagen does not increase after 3 weeks even though it continues to be synthesized and deposited at a rapid rate. Collagen is now being removed as quickly as it is formed (collagenolysis). The difference between the curves represents scar collagen turnover. (Reproduced by permission from Madden JW, Peacock EE Jr: Ann Surg 174:511, 1971)*

Approaches to the Control of Healing in Scar Tissue
Collagen synthesis
Collagen lysis
Collagen cross-linking

Apart from the beneficial effects of topical steroids,[28,29] attempts to alter synthetic and lytic activity have proven unsuccessful. The third technique, however, that of delaying collagen cross-linking, appears to be beneficial.[20,21,23] The main intermolecular bonds involve aldehyde groupings,[12,24] which can be effectively blocked with β-aminopro-prionitrile (BAPN) or penicillamine. Now, if the mechanical behavior of the resulting scar tissue is to be permanently altered, these changes at the molecular level must be reflected in an improved large-fiber organization. In penicillamine-treated wounds, minor but distinct improvements in collagen fiber aggregation have been demonstrated (Figs. 17 and 18).[30] The importance of these studies remains to be

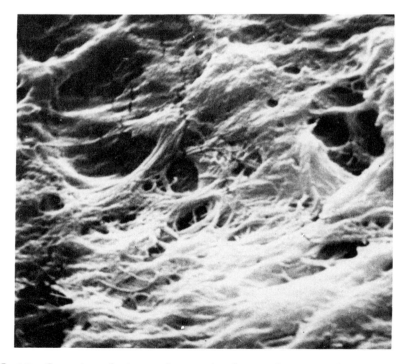

FIG. 17. *Scanning electron micrograph of a 20-day penicillamine-treated wound. The fibrils are forming into discrete bundles and a criss-cross pattern is suggested (×6400).*

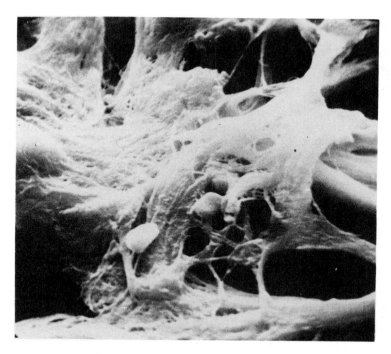

FIG. 18. *Scanning electron micrograph of a 60-day penicillamine-treated wound (×4200). The collagen fiber patterns are better organized than in the untreated wound (see Fig. 10). Large fibril bundles are well demarcated, and a network structure is developing.*

confirmed, but it does appear that collagen fiber patterns are improved when intermolecular cross-linking is temporarily delayed. This, in turn, may be associated with a more normal physical behavior of the scar. In particular, it is hoped that the wound will be stronger and less likely to contract pathologically.

SUMMARY

Wound healing is a pathological rather than a physiological process. The wound remains weak and brittle almost indefinitely. The abnormal physical behavior of scar tissue may result from abnormalities in the collagen fiber patterns within it. Temporarily delaying collagen cross-linking appears to encourage soft-tissue remodeling, and this may be associated with a closer approximation to the prewound state.

REFERENCES

1. Keill RH, Keitzer WF, Nichols WK, Henzel J, De Weese MS: Abdominal wound dehiscence. Arch Surg 106:573, 1973
2. Chvapil M: Pharmacology of fibrosis and tissue injury. Environ Health Perspect 9:283, 1974
3. Smith M, Enquist IF: A quantitative study of impaired healing resulting from infection. Surg Gynecol Obstet 125:965, 1967
4. Bentley JP: Rate of chondroitin sulfate formation in wound healing. Ann Surg 165:186, 1967
5. Forrest L, Jackson DS: Intermolecular cross-linking of collagen in human and guinea pig scar tissue. Biochim Biophys Acta 229:681, 1971
6. Jackson DS: The interaction of collagen with glycoproteins and proteoglycans. In Gibson T, van der Neulen JC (eds.): Wound Healing. Montreal, Foundation for International Cooperation in the Medical Sciences, 1975
7. Douglas DM: The healing of aponeurotic incisions. Br J Surg 40:79, 1952
8. Forrester JC, Zederfeldt BH, Hunt TK: A bioengineering approach to the healing wound. J Surg Res 9:207, 1969
9. Milch RA: Tensile strength of surgical wounds. J Surg Res 5:377, 1960
10. Douglas DM, Forrester JC, Ogilvie RR: Physical characteristics of collagen in the later stages of wound healing. Br J Surg 56:219, 1969
11. Dunphy JE, Udupa KN: Chemical and histochemical sequences in the normal healing of wounds. N Engl J Med 253:847, 1955
12. Grant ME, Prockop DJ: The biosynthesis of collagen. N Engl J Med 286:194, 242, 291, 1972
13. Miller EJ, Matukas VJ: Biosynthesis of collagen: The biochemist's view. Fed Proc 33:1197, 1974
14. Van Winkle W Jr: The tensile strength of wounds and factors that influence it. Surg Gynecol Obstet 129:819, 1969
15. Forrester JC, Zederfeldt BH, Hayes TL, Hunt TK: Mechanical biochemical and architectural features of repair. In Dunphy JE, Van Winkle W Jr (eds.), Repair and Regeneration. The Scientific Basis for Surgical Practice. New York, McGraw-Hill, 1969
16. Wolman M, Gillman T: A polarized light study of collagen in dermal wound healing. Br J Exp Pathol 53:85, 1972
17. Forrester JC, Hayes TL, Pease RFW, Hunt TK: Scanning electron microscopy of healing wounds. Nature 221:373, 1969
18. Brunius U, Zederfeldt B, Ahren C: Healing of skin incisions closed by non-suture technique: A tensiometric and histologic study in the rat. Acta Chir Scand 133:509, 1967
19. Forrester JC, Zederfeldt BH, Hayes TL, Hunt TK: Tape-closed and sutured wounds: A comparison by tensiometry and scanning electron microscopy. Br J Surg 57:729, 1970
20. Peacock EE Jr, Madden JW: Some studies on the effects of beta-aminoproprionitrile in patients with injured flexor tendons. Surgery 66:215, 1969
21. Peacock EE Jr, Madden JW: On the use of lathyrogens in human biology. Surgery 71:922, 1972
22. Chvapil M, Hurych J: Control of collagen biosynthesis. Int Rev Connect Tissue Res 4:67, 1968
23. Davis WM, Madden, JW, Peacock EE Jr: Nonoperative reversal of established esophageal stenosis. Surg Forum 23:399, 1972
24. Tanzer ML: Cross-linking of collagen. Science 180:561, 1973

25. Madden JW, Peacock EE Jr: Studies on the biology of collagen during wound healing. I. Rate of collagen synthesis and deposition in cutaneous wounds of the rat. Surgery 64:288, 1968

26. Madden JW, Peacock EE Jr: Studies on the biology of collagen during wound healing. III. Dynamic metabolism of scar collagen and remodeling of dermal wounds. Ann Surg 174:511, 1971

27. Riley WB Jr, Peacock EE Jr: Identification, distribution and significance of a collagenolytic enzyme in human tissues. Proc Soc Exp Biol Med 124:207, 1967

28. Berliner DJ, Williams RJ, Taylor GN, Nabors CJ Jr: Decreased scar formation with topical corticosteroid treatment. Surgery 61:619, 1967

29. Ketchum LD, Smith J, Robinson DW, Masters FW: The treatment of hypertrophic scar, keloid and scar contracture by triamcinolone acetonide. Plast Reconstr Surg 38:209, 1966

30. Forrester JC: Collagen fibre patterns in penicillamine treated wounds. A tensiometric and scanning electron microscope study. In Gibson T, van der Meulin JC (eds.): Wound Healing. Montreux, Foundation for International Cooperation in the Medical Sciences, 1975

Comment

One picture *is* worth a thousand words! To the best of my knowledge, Mr. Forrester was the first to turn the scanning electron microscope onto the healing wound. His photographs have added an immense dimension to our understanding of collagen deposition in wounds. In this chapter, however, Mr. Forrester does not discuss exactly how the new collagen "unites" the wound edges. New scanning views with collagen synthesis suppressed seem to show that collagen, the traditional constituent of glue, does just that! It "glues" the wound together by uniting to and surrounding the existing elements of the connective-tissue matrix.

Mr. Forrester took many of these photographs on one of Dr. Tom Hayes' earliest scanning scopes while the instrument was being developed in the University of California at Berkeley. His studies led us and many others to use this technique further. Most recently, we have photographed the effects of the collagen lytic process on colon collagen by suppressing collagen synthesis in experimental colon anastomoses.

Zinc and Other Factors of the Pharmacology of Wound Healing

11

M. Chvapil

This is a brief review of the present status of the pharmacology of fibrosis or wound healing. I will indicate some new trends and perspectives in the field. Unfortunately, achievements in the past 10 years, although theoretically valuable and exciting, are of questionable practical value to clinicians dealing with excessive wound healing in the form of hypertrophic scars, keloids, esophageal or urethral strictures, abdominal adhesions, or fibrotic lesions in general.[1]

SPECIFIC CONTROL OF COLLAGEN METABOLISM

The aim of this chapter is to answer a simple question: How efficiently can we control wound healing? Most research on wound healing has dealt with the products of fibroblast activity, namely, with collagen and glycosaminoglycans. If we look at the scheme of various aspects of collagen metabolism there exist several steps unique for collagen which could be used as a target for so-called "specific interference" with collagen metabolism.[2]

Scheme of Phases of Collagen Metabolism

Intracellular   Synthesis of collagenous polypeptide chain with additional (registering) peptides
Hydroxylation of proline and lysine residues
Glycosylation of ϵ-NH_2 of hydroxylysine
Secretion

Table 1. Methods of Specific Interference with Collagen Deposition

Metabolic Phase	Object	Mechanism of Interference	Pharmacologic Agent
Hydroxylation	Prolyl hydroxylase	Chelation of Fe^{++}, Fe^{+++}	1,10-phenanthroline, 2,2-dipyridyl desferrioxamine?
	Lysyl hydroxylase	Depletion of AscA	cis-4-hydroxy-L-proline L-azetidine-2-carboxylic acid
	Lysyl hydroxylase	Substrate modification	3,4-dehydro-L-proline cis-4-fluoro-L-proline trans-4,5-dehydro-L-lysine
Secretion	Microtubules	Degranulation	Colchicine
	Microfilaments	Degranulation	Vinblastin
Polymerization	Lysyl oxidase	Enzyme inhibition	BAPN systemic BAPN polymer—local
	Lysyl oxidase	Cu depletion during enzyme synthesis	Cu deficiency, high zinc treatment
	R-COH (aldehyde)	Complexing	D-penicillamine
	HC=N (Schiff base, nonreduced)	Cleavage of unstable cross-links	D-penicillamine
Degradation	Tissue collagenases	Enhanced synthesis	Colchicine
	Tissue collagenases	PMN cell infiltration	CaEDTA
Cell integrity	Fibrogenic cells	Agglutination or lysis	Antifibroblast serum

Extracellular Cleavage of additional peptides by procollagen peptidase

Polymerization or maturation of collagen by formation of intra- and intercellular covalent cross-links by lysyl oxidase

Degradation by collagenase (occurs at any stage of collagen life span, possibly intracellularly as well)

Some of these steps are hydroxylation of prolyl and lysyl residues by appropriate hydroxylases; glycosylation of some ϵ-NH$_2$ hydroxylysyl groups; the subsequent secretion of the molecule out of the cell; polymerization or maturation in the extracellular space under the effect of lysyl oxidase, which forms the basis for development of stable covalent cross-links; and degradation of the molecule, which may occur at any time and is perhaps faster in the younger molecules.

Let us analyze which of these reactions could be effectively controlled to such an extent that the final volume of deposited collagen or the physical characteristics of collagenous matrix in the injured tissue would be markedly changed.

Synthesis

The several methods by which one can interfere with various stages of collagen metabolism are summarized in Table 1. The hydroxylation of collagen could be limited by interference with ferrous iron or ascorbic acid cofactors of prolyl or lysyl hydroxylase or with divalent iron-chelating agents, or by limiting the supply of ascorbic acid, as is the case in scurvy. An ingenious method was proposed to render the newly formed collagen polypeptide chain resistant to hydroxylase by having incorporated into the polypeptide some nonhydroxylable proline or lysine analogs, such as azetidine-2-carboxylic acid, 4-6 cis-hydroxyproline, 3-4 dehydroproline, and 4-fluoroproline. In several elegant experiments carried on mainly by Prockop's group,[2] it was shown that by blocking hydroxylation of proline or lysine residues, such a molecule cannot be glycosylated and does not leave the fibroblast. Furthermore, underhydroxylated collagen is structurally unstable and is more susceptible to collagenase digestion. This was certainly one of the reasons such a research interest was paid to the control of collagen hydroxylation. Although these methods, represented by the chelation of Fe^{++}, ascorbic-acid control, or use of proline analogs, were able to limit collagen synthesis in in vitro systems (tissue slices, fibrogenic cells in tissue culture), they do not work in vivo.

Proline analogs in our hands were either toxic or ineffective.[3,4] There are several reasons for the inefficiency of proline analogs to block collagen synthesis in *in vivo* systems. It is difficult to reach sufficiently high concentrations of analogs in tissues to compete effectively with the rather large pool of free proline without inducing marked toxic effects on proteins other than collagen. Analogs are more toxic than proline (based on LD_{50}). Furthermore, the *t*-RNA has much higher affinity for proline than for analogs. Thus, only negligible amounts of analogs are incorporated into collagenous polypeptide *in vivo*. In summary, we do not know at the present time any acceptable method blocking the hydroxylation of collagen *in vivo*.

Chelating agents such as 2,2'-dipyridyl or 1,10-phenanthroline (to chelate iron) were able in some models of fibrosis (mainly in liver cirrhosis) to interfere with collagen deposition.[1] They work, however, by quite a different mechanism from the blocking of collagen hydroxylation. In fact, after a single injection of 1,10-phenanthroline in animals, the activity of prolyl hydroxylase in the skin or gut significantly rises (Fig. 1).[5] Low doses of 1,10-phenanthroline added to medium with fibroblasts significantly enhances prolyl hydroxylase activity as well, possibly by putting Fe^{++} into an "excited" state, in which oxygen is linked to this complex with higher affinity and efficiency.

Ascorbic-acid deficiency would be certainly a powerful method if we knew how to produce, in a defined and shorter time, a temporary

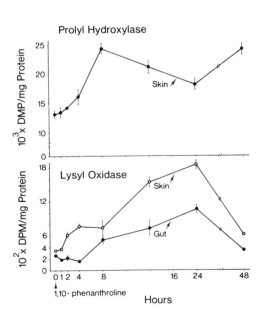

FIG. 1. In vivo administered 1,10-phenanthroline enhances the activity of prolyl hydroxylase and lysyl oxidase. 1,10-phenanthroline was administered to 60 g male rats at a dose of 2 mg/100 g as a single injection i.p. at various time intervals. Segments of the gut or skin were harvested for enzyme assay. There were 3 rats at each sampling period. Analyses done according to Chvapil et al. (Biochem Pharmacol 23:2165, 1974)

deficiency of this cofactor of prolyl hydroxylase.[6] In humans, it is un-predictable how quickly ascorbic-acid deficiency will develop.

Secretion

The cytoskeleton of the fibroblast consists of microtubules and micro-filaments and is involved in the transport and secretion of several pro-teins destined for transport.[2] Agents disintegrating the cytoskeletal structure of tubuline or actin and myosin would therefore block the secretion of collagen by the fibroblast. This again was shown nicely in a tissue-culture system of fibroblasts treated with the antitubular and antifilamentous agents colchicine, vinblastin, and cytochalasin B. Rojkind suggested that colchicine would effectively block collagen synthesis and deposition in vivo[7] and his group recently reported the successful use of colchicine in patients with rheumatoid arthritis.[8] Crit-ical evaluation of this method in animals as performed in our labora-tory[9,10] or in studies in humans as reported by Harris and co-workers[11] showed that colchicine is effective only at a dose which is quite toxic to animals. With such a dose, enhanced urinary excretion of hydrox-yproline parallels loss of body weight and enhanced tissue-collagenase activity in granuloma tissue and might be explained by a higher infil-tration of injured tissue by macrophages due to the cytotoxic effect of colchicine. In fact, Harris et al. did not observe any beneficial effect of colchicine in the treatment of rheumatoid arthritis.

Degradation

The exciting research in the field of collagen degradation by tissue collagenases is still not at a stage that would allow us to propose some practical method of enhancing collagen degradation in vivo by the activation of tissue collagenases. One aspect of collagen degradation related to collagenase of macrophages will be presented later.

Polymerization

The inhibition of maturation, or polymerization, of collagen has so far been the most successful and powerful pharmacological method inter-fering with physical properties of scar contractures and fibrotic stric-tures. It seems that it is not the total amount of collagen within a certain tissue, but rather the physical properties of the collagenous matrix which represent a real danger to the function of the tissue or organ (see Chapter 10). Only when collagen is cross-linked, possibly by stable covalent cross-links involving the function of lysyl oxidase, is it less degraded by collagenase and forms a compact, rigid scar. It is my belief that interference with the polymerization of collagen represents the only promising method in the field of pharmacology of wound healing at the present time.[1] In principle, we may interfere directly with the function of lysyl oxidase by various lathyrogenic agents, β-aminoproprionitrile (BAPN) being the most effective. Another possibility is to block the formed aldehydes, for instance by D-penicillamine, thus preventing the condensation of aldehydes or the formation of the Schiff bases, as shown in Figure 2. BAPN and D-penicillamine affect two different sites in the formation of covalent crosslinks and, thus, their effects are additive. One example of the efficacy of BAPN treatment has been tested not only in animal models of fibrosis, but also in two controlled human studies by Dr. Peacock and Dr. Madden in our unit. In testing the treatment of esophageal fibrotic stricture by BAPN,[12] we induced stenosis of the esophagus in dogs by chemical alkali injury. Four weeks after the injury was induced, when the inner diameter of the esophagus was reduced by approximately 70 percent, the treatment was begun and continued for 6 weeks. Without any treatment a stricture of esophagus persisted and resulted in enormous loss of weight through the 12-week observation period. When BAPN fumarate was administered intraperitoneally at a dose of 100 mg/kg body weight, the contracture of the scar was significantly less and the effect continued even after the BAPN administration was discontinued. The animal kept eating and contracture did not progress. These animals lived, without losing body weight, for 30 weeks. We believe that swallowed food dilated the injured area. At the same time, the collagen in the scar tissue of the esophagus of dogs treated with BAPN was much more soluble in both water and dilute saline than normal, evidence of established lathyrism (poorly connected collagen fibers).

Although lysyl oxidase is a copper-containing enzyme, copper chelators are ineffective in blocking its activity. In dietary copper deficiency, however, lysyl oxidase activity was diminished, and collagen or elastin extractability was increased. Because of the known antagonism of copper and zinc, it is possible to induce copper deficiency by feeding a high-zinc diet, and we found inhibition of lysyl oxidase in granuloma tissue by administration of high doses of zinc to rats.[13] This, however, should not be considered a feasible method for humans, because of possible problems with administering high doses of zinc.

There is much more convincing evidence about the high efficacy of BAPN administered in vivo on the physical characteristics of collagenous structures.[14] In our experiments,[15] we observed that a dose significantly lower than that required to induce the changes in collagen

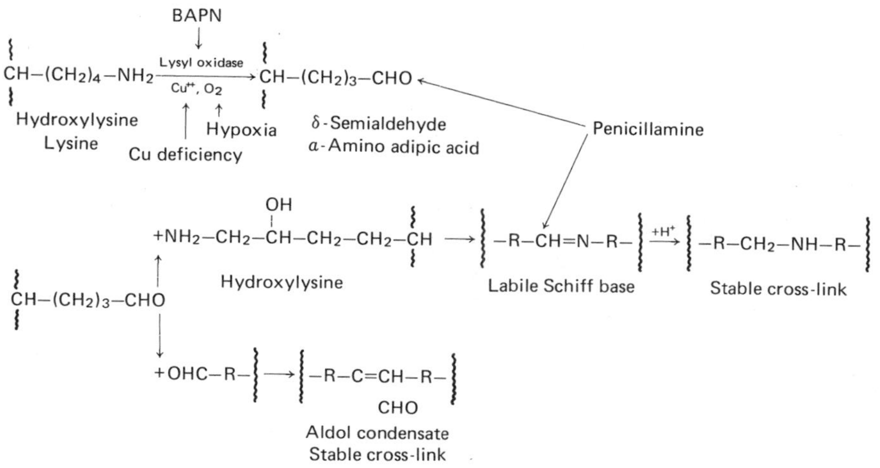

FIG. 2.   *Control of covalent cross-linking in collagen. β-Aminoproprionitrile (BAPN) irreversibly links to lysyl oxidase, which is also inhibited in copper-deficient states. If hypoxia inhibits lysyl oxidase directly, as indicated by our previous work, it remains to be proven. D-penicillamine binds to aldehydes formed by the oxidative deamination of ϵ-NH$_2$ groups of lysine and hydroxylysine by lysyl oxidase, thus preventing these groups from forming either stable aldol condensate or Schiff bases. D-penicillamine also cleaves the non-reduced (still unstable) Schiff bases, thus increasing the portion of "extractable collagens."*

extractability and physical characteristics of collagen (5–10 mg BAPN/ 100 g body weight/day) will almost completely inhibit lysyl oxidase. Still, such a low dose does not affect the solubility or extractability of collagen to such an extent as the higher dose (50–100 mg). Therefore, we believe that at the higher doses needed for therapeutic effect we not only inhibit lysyl oxidase, and thus prevent the formation of cross-links, but there is also a secondary effect of BAPN which may possibly consist in activation of collagenolytic mechanisms and which would thus contribute to an increased pool of soluble collagen and decrease physical strength of the collagenous tissue. This is under investigation. It is also interesting that after a single dose of BAPN, the enzyme activity was inhibited for approximately 6 hours. After 24 hours, the enzyme had regained the activity. This indicates either an enormous capacity to synthesize the enzyme *de novo* or that the linkage of BAPN with lysyl oxidase is reversible. In summary, interference with collagen polymerization by lathyrogens, mainly BAPN, seems so far to be the only effective method of controlling the characteristics of the collagenous structures in the wound or fibrotic tissue.

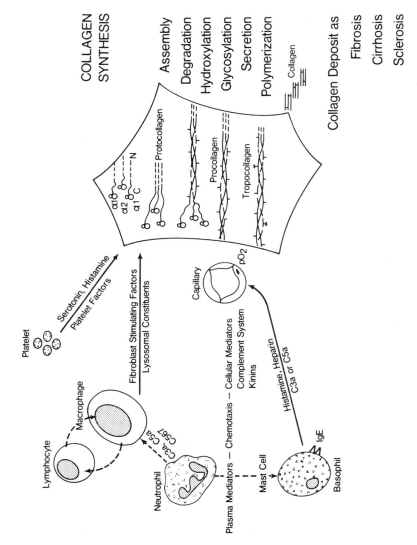

FIG. 3.   *Highly simplified scheme of the cellular aspects of fibroproliferative inflammation.*

CONTROL OF THE PROLIFERATIVE PHASE
(CELLULAR ASPECT)

There are several other approaches to the control of wound healing. We have to keep in mind that wound healing is based on an inflammatory process and, therefore, that several events occur before the fibroblast becomes activated. Figure 3 schematically illustrates the hierarchy of reactions where, because of physical, chemical, or biological noxious agents, cell activators and mediators of inflammation are released, bringing into the injured area cells like polymorphonuclear leukocytes (which release lysosomal enzymes, modify complement components 3 to 5 to form anaphylatoxins, and produce some other factors stimulating macrophages), basophils, eosinophils, and platelets. A review of these aspects of the inflammatory reaction in healing wounds is presented at this symposium by Ross (Chapter 1) and Hunt et al. (Chapter 22). There certainly exists an exciting dialogue between inflammatory cells, but not every cell talks to the other. Some cells communicate directly, some indirectly. Many of these cells have the capacity, when activated, to promote the activity of fibroblasts. This topic is beautifully discussed in Chapter 1. At the same time, substances such as histamine and serotonin change the microcirculation. Hypoxia is a common part of the inflammatory lesion and may be another factor both promoting and limiting fibroblast activity. This is, however, a very controversial topic and let me make reference to such experts as Drs. Silver, Niinikoski, and Hunt (Chapters 2, 5, and 22). This complex reaction has been the object of treatment with various anti-inflammatory drugs, antihistamines, antiserotonin drugs, and so on.

ZINC AS AN ANTI-INFLAMMATORY DRUG

The effect of zinc on the reactivity of various inflammatory cells is the topic my laboratory has been involved in during the last four years, and we have presented evidence indicating that the activity of polymorphonuclear leukocytes, macrophages, platelets in addition to mast cells, as shown by Uvnas and Hogberg and by Kazimierrzak and Maslinski, are inhibited by in vitro or in vivo administration of large amounts of zinc.[16,17,18] Zinc seems to be involved in cell homeostasis. Thus, the phagocytosis, bacterial killing, chemotaxis, and O_2 consumption of activated polymorphonuclear leukocytes is inhibited by the addition of zinc ions to the medium. Peritoneal macrophages isolated from animals kept on a high-zinc diet or treated with zinc parenterally show less motility. They are rather rounded as compared with the active macrophages with several elongations and extrusions of the protoplasmic membrane. Release of serotonin or aggregability of platelets, which are rightfully considered inflammatory cells, are also inhibited in the presence of large amounts of zinc ions. We have been involved in studying the mechanism of zinc's effect on the cell activity and, although we already have some data pointing to the possible mode of zinc effect on cells, I rather prefer to postulate a general working scheme indicating that zinc might interfere with some functional groups at the membrane level such as with the phosphate group of phospholipids, carboxyl groups of sialoprotein, or sulfhydryl groups of protein. Zinc might block some enzymes controlling the fluidity of the membrane, like phospholipase A_2 or ATPase in general. Zinc may also interfere with NADPH oxidation by direct linking to this pyridine nucleotide although this is uncertain. It is plausible to assume (because of the known antagonism of Zn and Cu) that Zn^{++} may displace Cu^{++} required for the function and integrity of cell microskeleton. Finally, it is worth mentioning that superoxide dismutase is a zinc metalloenzyme which contributes to the maintenance of the intracellular organell's integrity by scavenging superoxide and singlet oxygen.

The functional immobilization of some inflammatory cells by large amounts of zinc does not mean that the well-known positive effect of zinc on wound healing is related to any of the mechanisms already discussed. The evidence is still lacking in spite of my personal view that, in those wounds that heal by excessive scar formation, too many inflammatory cells collect and too high a turnover rate of these cells (activation-release of activators, lysosomal enzymes, cell death, etc.) might be a major reason for this undesirable "superhealing." This raises again the question of the role of macrophages in fibroproliferative reactions, as already discussed at this symposium by Dr. Ross (Chapter 1).

ZINC AND WOUND HEALING

Now, how to explain the enhancement of wound healing by zinc shown by several authors? I personally do not believe that the administration of zinc enhances wound healing above the normal rate of healing process as it occurs in nutritionally well-balanced persons.[19] Our experiments with zinc and the activity of inflammatory cells show that in the zinc-deficient state the activity of cells like macrophages or polymorphonuclear leukocytes is enhanced as compared with the normal zinc-saturated animals. This would indicate to me that in zinc-deficient subjects (or those low in zinc) most surgical wounds heal under slightly abnormal influx of polymorphonuclear leukocytes and macrophages, which cause more necrosis, more debridement, and rather uncontrolled lesions. In addition, the activity of several enzymes essential for cell reproduction, such as DNA polymerase and reverse transcriptase, are Zn metalloenzymes. By limiting inflammatory cell reaction or proliferation, by zinc, for instance, we might control the rate of wound healing. It seems that the optimal rate of wound healing occurs in nutritionally well-balanced persons or animals. We have to keep in mind that there are many situations under which the patient becomes zinc deficient. It is the chronicity of injury, repetitive stress, and various hormones such as ACTH, corticoids, progesterone, and estrogens (oral contraceptives) that decrease the zinc content of the body (in addition to intestinal fistulae, diarrhea, etc.). In those patients with subnormal biological zinc levels, problems in wound healing may be corrected by peroral supplementation of zinc.[20,21,22]

ANTIMACROPHAGE AND ANTIFIBROBLAST SERUM AND WOUND HEALING

The degree of fibrotic change in a certain tissue (referring mainly to liver and lung) depends on the extent of necrosis within the lesion. The macrophage is the major cell involved in removing the cell debris. At the same time, however, activated macrophages produce substances known to stimulate either mitosis of fibroblasts, as discussed in Chapter 1 and 22, or activity of fibroblasts, as shown in Table 2, referring

Table 2. Antisera Effect on Granuloma Tissue*

Treatment	Collagen Synthesis (cpm/μg Hyp)	Prolyl Hydroxylase (cpm/μg DNA)
Antimacrophage	41.4± 4.4	22.7±1.4
Antithymocyte	71.8±11.3	30.8±3.2
Normal serum	64.4±10.0	30.0±2.7
Saline	67.6± 8.9	31.8±4.7

* Sera against rat peritoneal macrophages and thymocytes prepared as indicated in Table 3. Rats treated by a procedure similar to that outlined in Table 3 for 14 days. Data refer to analysis of granuloma tissue formed as reaction to subcutaneous implanted Ivalon PVA sponges. Presented as X ± SEM. Only rats treated with AMS showed a significant slower rate of collagen synthesis and less activity of prolyl hydroxylase in the granuloma tissue. (Steinbronn D, Steinbronn K, Chvapil M: unpublished data)

to one of our own experiments. Similar evidence has been presented by several other authors. Thus, it seems that by reducing or limiting the participation of macrophages in fibroproliferative inflammation or in the repair process, less collagen would be deposited in the form of a scar. This was in fact nicely shown by Leibovich and Ross,[23] who treated guinea pig wounds with antimacrophage serum (AMS) and showed, by morphometric methods, a reduction in collagen fiber formation within the wound. In our experiments, performed by Del and Karen Steinbronn and myself, we prepared antimacrophage serum against rat peritoneal macrophages and administered this rather monocyte-specific serum daily to rats with implanted polyvinyl-alcohol sponges for a total of 12 days. A significant reduction in the rate of collagen biosynthesis as well as in prolyl hydroxylase activity in granuloma tissue of treated rats was found in comparison with control rats, treated either with saline, normal saline, or antithymocyte serum (see Table 2). Morphological analysis suggested lesser infiltration of the lesion with macrophages.

We also tested and described the first experience with antifibroblast serum (AFS) effect on collagen synthesis in granuloma tissue.[24] The results (Table 3) showed a significant decrease in prolyl hydroxylase activity and collagen content in granuloma of animals treated with AFS. The use of AMS or AFS in the control of collagen synthesis and deposition indicates a potential method of controlling scarring. Still, at the present time, it is more academic than practical.

Table 3. Antifibroblast Serum Effect on Granuloma Tissue in Balb-cJ Mice*

Treatment	Sponge Dry Weight (mg ± SEM)	Collagen (hyp mg/g ± SEM)	Prolyl Hydroxylase (cpm/mg DNA ± SEM)
Saline	23.5 ± 1.6	2.6 ± 0.45	
Homologous serum	32.5 ± 1.0†	3.3 ± 0.30	63.7 ± 7.1
Antifibroblast serum	35.9 ± 3.3	1.9 ± 0.58‡	27.2 ± 3.2§

* Antiserum was prepared against Balb-cJ mouse fibroblasts, injected into rabbits with Freund's complete adjuvant till titer 1:1024 was obtained. Harvested antiserum was decomplemented, absorbed with Balb-cJ mouse-formed blood cells to remove all common and cross-reacting cellular antibodies. Three groups of 6 Balb-cJ mice each were implanted with two polyvinyl-alcohol sponges per mouse. Each mouse received daily intraperitoneal injections with 0.3 ml/kg of either saline, homologous rabbit serum, or AFS for 12 consecutive days. (After Steinbronn D, Carlson EC, Chvapil M: Surg Forum 25:44, 1974)

†p<.01; ‡p<.05; §p<.001.

CONTROL OF LIPID PEROXIDATION

Research of recent years indicates that the magnitude of peroxidation of polyunsaturated fatty-acid constituents of various cell membranes depends on the degree of activity of the cell or tissue and the balance between oxidative stimuli and the concentration of antioxidants or free-radical scavengers. Thus, in active cells like macrophages or platelets, a higher formation of lipid peroxides has been shown. In inflamed tissue, there is higher formation of malondialdehyde or fluorescent products as evidence of lipid peroxidation. Enhanced lipid peroxidation indicates higher breakdown of tissue cell-membrane-bounded compartments as disintegrated lysosomal vacuoles break and release lysosomal enzymes, as the endoplasmic reticulum loses the capacity to synthesize proteins, and as mitochondria lose the capacity for oxidative phosphorylation. The control of lipid peroxidation of free-radical scavengers like vitamin E; the direct protection against the effect of free radicals by protecting the activity of glutathione peroxidase by selenium; the enhancement of superoxide dismutase (a Zn enzyme) or of the content of reducing components such as glutathione or cysteine and, eventually, ascorbic acid might explain the effectiveness of these drugs on the rate of wound healing. This highly simplified outline of lipid peroxidation as the mechanism of tissue injury, wound healing included, has become a very fruitful working hypothesis to understand some events of wound healing.[25,26]

CONTROL OF THE INTEGRITY OF BIOMEMBRANES

One cannot doubt the importance of the integrity of biological membranes and cells in the normal process of wound healing. Any factor disintegrating the membrane will ultimately result in modification of the healing process. This might be the mechanism of the effect of vitamin A. At low levels, vitamin A incorporates into the biological membranes, dissolves in the lipid moiety, and contributes to the integrity of the membrane. At larger doses, however, vitamin A in the membrane seems to contribute to its disintegration. This mechanism was proposed by Dingle[27] to explain the effect of vitamin A in developing rheumatoid arthritis. I wonder if the same holds for skin wounds. At the appropriate pole of this category belong the effects of corticoids and several antirheumatoid and anti-inflammatory agents and, according to our preliminary results, also zinc. All of those agents tend to stabilize lysosomal membranes.

In summary, I would stress that there certainly exists a whole battery of methods for controlling individual steps and features of the wound-healing process. Only a few methods are established and documented to such an extent that they could be successfully used in humans. More basic research, therefore, is needed to "master" wound healing so that surgeons will be in the fortunate position of knowing how to control hypertrophic scar or keloids and, eventually, other forms of fibrotic or cirrhotic lesions in humans.

REFERENCES

1. Chvapil M: Pharmacology of fibrosis: Definitions, limits and perspectives. Life Sci 16:1345, 1975
2. Grant ME, Prockop DJ: The biosynthesis of collagen. N Engl J Med 286:195, 1972
3. Chvapil M, McCarthy D, Madden JW, Peacock EE Jr: Effect of cishydroxyproline on collagen and other proteins in skin wounds, granuloma tissue and liver of mice and rats. Exp Mol Pathol 20:363, 1974
4. Madden JW, Chvapil M, Carlson EC, Ryan JN: Toxicity and metabolic effects of 3,4-dehydroproline in mice. Toxicol Appl Pharmacol 26:426, 1973
5. Chvapil M, McCarthy D, Madden JW, Peacock EE Jr: Effect of 1,10-phenanthroline and desferrioxamine in vivo in prolyl hydroxylase and hydroxylation of collagen in various tissues in rats. Biochem Pharmacol 23:2165, 1974
6. Barnes MJ, Kodicek E: Biological hydroxylations and ascorbic acid with special regard to collagen metabolism. Vitam Horm 30:1, 1972
7. Rojkind M, Kershenobich D: Effect of colchicine on collagen, albumin and transferrin synthesis by cirrhotic rat liver slices. Biochim Biophys Acta 378:415, 1975
8. Alarcon-Sergovia D, Ibanez G, Kershenobich D, Rojkind M: Treatment of scleroderma. Lancet 1:1054, 1974
9. Morton D Jr, Steinbronn K, Lato M, Chvapil M, Peacock EE: Effect of colchicine on wound healing in rats. Surg Forum 25:27, 1974
10. Blau S, Peacock EE Jr, Carlson EC, Chvapil M: Effect of colchicine on crosslinking of collagen in rats. Surg Forum 26:5, 1975
11. Harris ED Jr, Hoffman GS, McGuire JL, Strosberg JM: Colchicine: Effects upon urinary hydroxyproline excretion in patients with scleroderma. Metabolism 24:529, 1975
12. Madden JW, Davis WM, Butler C, Peacock EE Jr: Experimental esophageal lye burns II. Correcting established strictures with beta-aminopropionitrile and bougienage. Ann Surg 178:277, 1973
13. Chvapil M, Stankova L, Weldy P, Bernhard D, Campbell J, Carlson EC, Cox T, Peacock J, Bartos Z, Zukowki C: The role of zinc in the function of some inflammatory cells. In Brewer GJ, Prasad AS (eds): Zinc Metabolism: Current Aspects in Health and Disease. New York, Liss, 1977
14. Peacock EE: Biology of wound repair. Life Sci 13,4:i–ix, 1973

15. Arem A, Madden JW, Chvapil M, Tillema L: Effect of lysyl oxidase inhibition of healing wounds. Surg Forum 26:67, 1975
16. Chvapil M: New aspects in the biological role of zinc: A stabilizer of macromolecules and biological membranes. Life Sci 13:1041, 1973
17. Chvapil M, Elias SL, Ryan JN, Zukoski CF: Pathophysiology of zinc. In Pfeiffer CS (ed): International Review of Neurobiology. New York, Academic Press, 1972
18. Chvapil M, Zukoski CF, Hattler BG, Stankova L, Montgomery D, Carlson EC, Ludwig JC: Zinc and cells. In Prasad AS (ed): Trace Elements in Human Health and Disease. New York, Academic Press, 1976
19. Elias S, Chvapil M: Zinc and wound healing in normal and chronically ill rats. J Surg Res 15:59, 1973
20. Halsted JA, Smith JC Jr, Irwin MI: A conspectus of research on zinc requirements of man. J Nutr 104:345, 1974
21. Burch RE, Hahn HKJ, Sullivan JF: Newer aspects of the roles of zinc, manganese, and copper in human nutrition. Clin Chem 21:501, 1975
22. Chesters JK: Biochemical functions of zinc in animals. World Rev Nutr Diet 32:135, 1978
23. Leibovich SJ, Ross R: The role of the macrophage in wound repair. Am J Pathol 78:71, 1975
24. Steinbronn D, Carlson EC, Chvapil M: Antifibroblast serum: A new method of controlling collagen synthesis. Surg Forum 25:44, 1974
25. Barber AA, Bernheim F: Lipid peroxidation: its measurement, occurrence, and significance in animal tissues. Adv Gerontol Res 2:355, 1967
26. Tappel AL: Lipid peroxidation damage to cell components. Fed Proc 32:1970, 1973
27. Dingle JT, Lucy JA: Vitamin A, carotenoids and cell function. Biol Rev 40:422, 1965

Comment

Dr. Chvapil's summary of methods by which wound healing and scarring may be controlled spans the efforts of the past, the present, and probably the future. He is, of course, thinking pharmacologically. As he points out, his comments should be taken in the context of many other chapters in this book. The implications of his comments taken in the light of Chapters 1, 2, 5, 11, 21, and 22 test the ability of one's imagination to comprehend.

Dr. Chvapil, and the rest of us, have not mentioned two well-established means of controlling repair: corticosteroids and pressure and traction. In addition, we have given nutrition a sort of passing nod. Steroids, of course, are not directly related to repair in most people's eyes. However, steroids combine with cell receptors in macrophages to reduce the secretion of various enzymes, reduce motility, reduce chemotaxis, and interfere seriously with the ability of the organism to mount the inflammatory response which is so important to repair. This may be, to the minds of medical people, a side effect of steroids; but it is more than a side effect to a patient on steroids who cannot heal. Traction and pressure, a method developed and popularized by Larson, Bauer, and others, has been particularly effective in the treatment of contractures due to burns and chronic scarring or inflammation around joints. This is a powerful and well-established method in which physical force can be channeled to stretch the plastic collagen fibers, influence their reconstruction through biological forces as yet unknown, and reduce their mass through the lysis of collagen and limitation of blood supply.

Many of the concepts Dr. Chvapil has dealt with are difficult to express because of the simple rule that there may be too much of a good thing. For instance, consider the dilemma of zinc. Zinc deficiency impairs a number of enzymes, including superoxide dismutase. The "proper" amount of zinc keeps us functioning normally, but no one knows if the normal zinc content is adequate for an injured patient. Zinc can be "toxic," but so can therapeutic doses of steroids be "toxic." We merely accept the toxicity of the substance as a desirable compromise under the circumstances. Therefore, the ideal amount of zinc probably varies from what we might normally consider too little to too much. Iron, for instance, the staff of life in adequate quantities, can be poisonous in larger quantities. Dr. Chvapil brings up the question of whether large doses of zinc may become therapeutic in the patient who threatens to develop hypertrophic scar. This will be a difficult question to answer. As he points out, large doses of zinc appear to be relatively safe until they begin to deplete the body of copper. To avoid such a systemic complication, one thinks of topical application. Is it possible that my mother, who put zinc oxide on all my wounds, was doing me a favor after all?

In the section on lipid peroxidation, Dr. Chvapil is looking into a very dim future. Although it is dim, I have one of those gut feelings that says that behind the clouds there may be a number of beautiful vistas. For instance, there is a developing idea that white cells aggregate in capillaries as a result of toxemia or trauma, even distant trauma. These white cells seem to be "activated"; and when they are "activated," they use major amounts of oxygen and convert it to major amounts of high-energy free radicals of oxygen, including superoxide, hydroxyl radical, singlet oxygen, and others. When the white cell sticks to the endothelial cell of the capillary, an area of high oxidation-reduction potential may result, much to the detriment of the endothelium. When oxygen is in good supply, as in the lung, this could be a potent means of injury to vascular endothelium. Is it possible, then, that the use of free-radical scavengers might protect humans against some aspects of organ failure? Manitol has protected against pulmonary failure after injury and is a free-radical scavenger. In wounds, on the other hand, the white cell needs the free radicals to kill bacteria. The fibroblast needs them to synthesize and hydroxylate collagen. Superoxide and other radicals have a definite and constructive role. Yet cell membrane integrity is important to wounds.

Again, we must seek a balance. The vascular injury of wounded tissues prevents oxygen delivery to such an extent that it seems impossible to overoxygenate wounds at atmospheric pressures. In fact, it appears desirable to increase their oxygenation in many cases. The challenge is to increase the oxygenation of the wound without overoxygenating some other part of the body.

The pharmacological control of repair is fraught with this kind of difficulty. One person's meat is still another's poison. The resuscitative fluid therapy we give today to save the lives of burned patients may become their pulmonary edema tomorrow. The questions are complex but the same is true of many drugs used for the support and manipulation of the vascular system. In that case, with the profusion of means by which we can measure physiology, we can use the minute-by-minute requirements for vasodilators, vasoconstrictors, and cardiotonic agents and discontinue or increase them as the signs of more or less need or more or less toxicity are detected. We hope that circumstances can become similar for control of scar. The basic need would seem to be to develop means of measuring cellular activity in wounds that will allow us to detect early the trends to excessive or inadequate function of reparative cells.

Colon Repair: The Collagenous Equilibrium

12

T. K. Hunt, P. R. Hawley, J. Hale, W. Goodson, and K. K. Thakral

One of the main concepts to have arisen in Dr. Dunphy's laboratories, and among those of us who have worked with him, is that of the balance between collagen synthesis and lysis in wound healing. For many years, we emphasized the importance of collagen synthesis in wounds without recognizing the simple fact that, if collagen could be made as rapidly as it seems, lysis would be a necessary mechanism to protect us from being frozen in our own connective tissues. About 1960, several investigators recognized that collagen lytic manifestations are all around us.

Surgeons might have noted as examples of collagen lysis how retention sutures cut though tissue or how indurated scars soften. The observation that finally "stuck," however, was that of Gross and Lapierre, who noted that the collagen in a tadpole's tail had to be lysed to allow the tadpole to become a frog![1] They pursued this observation and isolated an extracellular enzyme now called *collagenase*. The source of this enzyme and its environmental requirements have since become a matter of considerable debate. Whether it is the only enzyme that can cleave collagen into products susceptible to other proteases has also been controversial. At the moment, it appears that fibroblasts and leukocytes release collagenase. Collagenases may be more or less permanently attached to collagen fibers where they are activated by certain physiologic or biochemical events to exercise their latent lytic activity. It also appears that collagenase is not the only enzyme which lyses collagen. A number of so-called lysozomal enzymes can cleave collagen in the extracellular space. The biologic importance of the collagenase versus the lysozomal enzymes is still under debate.

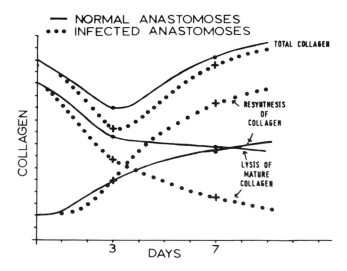

FIG. 1. Collagen synthesis and lysis as measured by hydroxyproline incorporation (synthesis) and decrease of specific activity of prelabeled collagen (lysis) in colon anastomosis in animals. Since the two measurements are expressed in different units, the ordinate units are not labeled and no direct comparisons are valid; but the conflicting trends are obvious. Lysis is far more active and lasts longer in infected anastomoses. In this experiment, the infected anastomoses synthesized collagen. Infection sometimes stimulates and sometimes may retard synthesis. When synthesis is retarded, lysis proceeds unbalanced with disastrous results. (From Hawley[6])

Cronin, Jackson, and Dunphy were the first to point out that a major collagen lysis occurs in the area of a colon anastomosis.[2,3] Their original estimate was that 50 percent of the pre-existing collagen in the few millimeters surrounding an anastomosis of the colon in a rat is lysed by the end of the first week after anastomosis. This estimate may have proved slightly large, but the effect is a major biologic phenomenon to a surgeon! It demonstrates that, in a very real sense, the integrity of an anastomosis becomes a race between the tendency of the inflammatory reaction to lyse old collagen and the ability of fibroblasts to make new collagen. Figure 1 shows this balance.[4,5,6] To measure lysis in these studies, Dr. Hawley labeled the normal collagen of young animals with radioactive proline during the growth period. A colon anastomosis was made months later. After colon anastomosis, pieces of nearby colon were removed and residual radioactivity was compared with that from similarly treated animals that were not operated upon. Other animals were given radioactive proline after injury, and the accumulation of radioactive hydroxyproline in the anastomosis is shown as a measure of wound collagen synthesis. Figure 1 strikingly demonstrates the balance between synthesis and lysis. The tensile integrity of the suture line, which is roughly proportional to the total collagen content, obviously depends upon synthesis staying ahead of lysis.

There is a very murky area involving which of the collagens, the new or the old, is lysed and how much of each. It is impossible, at this time, to estimate exactly how much collagen is lysed and carried away except that it is a clinically significant amount. It is perhaps not important, however, to make the distinction between lysis of new or old collagen in patients, since the suture is not discriminating about which type of collagen it leans on in order to hold the tissues together. However, Jiborn and Zederfeldt have shown the balance to be far more precarious in the proximal colon segment where dilation may become a problem postoperatively (unpublished data).

Mr. Irvin (Chapter 13) re-examined the balance between collagen synthesis and lysis, using rather more precise techniques than were available to either Cronin, Jackson, and Dunphy or Hawley, Hale, and Hunt. He showed that the lysis of old collagen in the animal colon anastomosis may be closer to 25 percent[7] than the 50 percent estimated by Cronin et al.[2] Experiments from our laboratory by Hale tend to support the lower estimate.[8] Hale also showed how fragile the process of collagen synthesis is (Fig. 2). This information was obtained by the

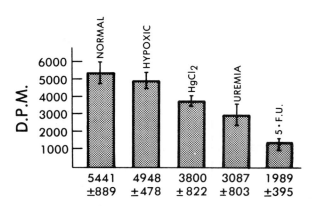

FIG. 2. *Collagen synthesis as measured by the H^3-proline-specific activity of collagen soluble in neutral 0.4 N saline found in tissue taken from animal colon anastomoses at 7 days. The H^3 proline was injected 24 hours prior to sampling of tissue and is thus an approximation of collagen synthesis. $HgCl_2$ has been used especially in Great Britain as a tumoricidal wash of the open colon during colectomy. The animals given 5-fluorouracil were obviously ill during its administration. We would expect the effect to be dose-related. (From Hale[8])*

same methods used by Hawley.[6] Clearly, chemical damage done during operation ($HgCl_2$ is often used as a tumoricidal wash in colectomies) is harmful, as is chemotherapy. Hypoxia (rather mild in this case) seems not as harmful to colon repair as it is to skin or bone healing (see Chapter 5). There is no ready explanation for this difference, but it agrees with Irvin's results. Synthesis is an energy-consuming process and is more labile than is lysis, which tends to occur almost without regard to the patient's physiology except that it is greatly enhanced by infection and starvation. Lysis, therefore, is always a "threat," and one must insure, somehow, that collagen synthesis is supported. As Figure 3 shows, the trauma of a laparotomy is enough to activate collagen lysis in the entire gastrointestinal tract.

Recently, we have managed to find microscopic evidence of the collagenous equilibrium in rabbit colon anastomoses. Although this does not represent a systematic inquiry, scanning electron photomicrographs of submucosa of normal colon (Fig. 4) contrast markedly with those from a colon anastomosis in a rabbit subjected to repeated operative stress and hypovolemia (Fig.5). A specimen taken from a normally healing anastomosis is shown in Figure 6. Re-examination of Figure 5 now shows so obviously the appearance of scar collagen (Fig. 6) and the lysis of old collagen (Fig. 5).

Despite the debates over details, we feel that this concept, that an-

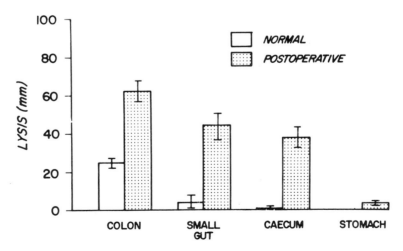

FIG. 3.   *Measurement of collagen lysis capacity in the mucosa and submucosa of animal colon. Fresh specimens of tissue, precisely weighed, were placed on native collagen gel under culture fluid and the circle of clarity in the normally opalescent collagen gel was measured. The size of this circle is a rough but useful measure of lytic capacity.*

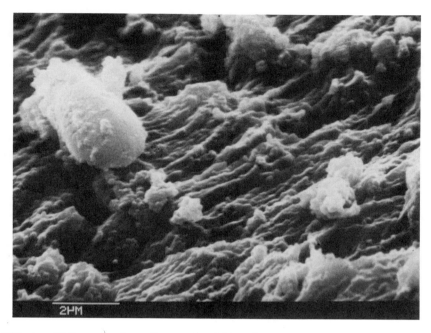

FIG. 4.   Oblique section of normal rabbit submucosa at × 20,000 under the scanning electron microscope. Human submucosa is similar. The collagen fibrils are arranged in sheets and bands.

astomotic integrity is a race between collagen synthesis and lysis, is one of the most compelling and useful concepts we can bring to the surgical patient. It brings a sense of haste to physiological and nutritional support. It adds to the concept of inflammatory collagen lysis given by Mr. Irvin in the next chapter. It brings an urgency to the control of contamination, to gentle surgery, and to physiological support. More than anything, it gives us the feeling that we have the means to minimize suture-line leaks. The kind of discipline that this concept has engendered has allowed several surgical centers to lower clinically apparent anastomotic leak rates in colon surgery to the level of approximately 2 percent. Obviously, that figure can be confounded by patient selection as Mr. Irvin's chapter shows. However, the very concept of collagen balance allows us, as Dr. Schrock will show (Chapter 14), to make sounder judgments in selecting patients for colostomy or anastomosis.

The last results of this line of reasoning are not yet in. Hawley et al. have shown that collagenase has its inhibitor or inhibitors in serum, as do many enzymes.[9] He found a suggestion that there may be con-

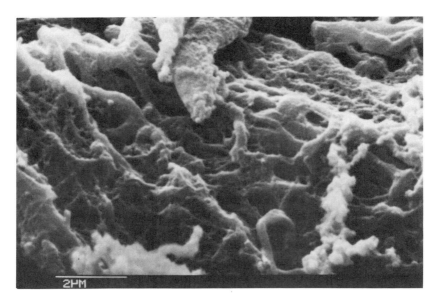

FIG. 5. Submucosa (× 20,000) taken from a colon anastomosis in an animal which had been operated twice during 7 days and had moderate peritonitis. It was clinically ill. Note the lacunae "eaten" in the sheets of collagen and compare with Figure 4.

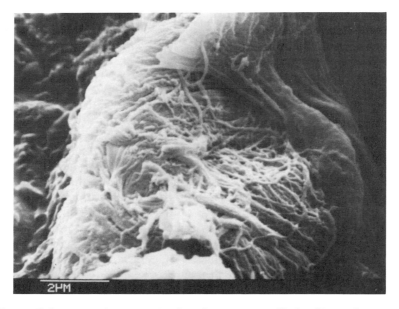

FIG. 6. Submucosa (× 20,000) taken from a normally healing colon anastomosis. Note the new, finely fibrillar, rather irregular collagen which is deposited on the edges of partially lysed collagen fibers. Compare with Figures 3 and 4.

stitutional differences in these inhibitors and, therefore, major variations in rates of lysis between patients. Obviously, a slowing of local
lysis could have enormous benefit for the occasional patient. Unfortunately, the lytic mechanisms have proved difficult to study, and it
is not yet time to manipulate collagen lysis in surgical patients. When
the concept can be applied, it may become extremely important to the
surgeon.

REFERENCES

1. Gross J, Lapiere CM: Collagenolytic activity in amphibian tissues: a tissue
   culture assay. Proc Natl Acad Sci USA 48:1014, 1962
2. Cronin K, Jackson DS, and Dunphy JE: Changes in bursting strength and
   collagen content of the healing colon. Surg Gynecol Obstet 126:747, 1968
3. Conin K, Jackson DS, Dunphy JE: Specific activity of hydroxyproline-trit-
   ium in the healing colon. Surg Gynecol Obstet 126:1061, 1968
4. Hunt TK, Hawley PR: Surgical judgment and colonic anastomoses. Dis
   Colon Rectum 12:167, 1969
5. Hawley PR, Hunt TK, Dunphy, JE: Aetiology of colonic anastomotic leaks.
   Proc Soc Med [Suppl] 63:28, 1970
6. Hawley PR: The aetiology of colonic anastomotic leaks with specific reference to the role of collagenase. Master's Thesis, University of London,
   1969
7. Irvin TT, Hunt TK: Reappraisal of the healing process of anastomosis of
   the colon. Surg Gynecol Obstet 138:741, 1974
8. Hale JE: The effect of cytotoxic solutions on suture-line tumor recurrence
   and on healing of colon anastomosis. Master's Thesis, University of London, 1976
9. Hawley PR, Faulk WP, Hunt TK, Dunphy JE: Collagenase activity in the
   gastrointestinal tract. Br J Surg 57:896, 1970

Problems of Repair in the Colon: Laboratory and Clinical Correlations

13

Thomas T. Irvin

Disruption of a colonic anastomosis is a serious complication and is accompanied by a significant mortality. In a study of 203 colonic anastomoses (Irvin and Goligher 1973), there was an operative mortality of 6.5 percent, and almost all of this mortality resulted from anastomotic dehiscence. Clinical evidence of dehiscence occurred in 14 percent of cases, and the true incidence of dehiscence was probably higher. Careful examination of anastomoses in the left colon or rectum by a postoperative barium or gastrografin enema not infrequently shows a defect in the anastomosis which is not apparent clinically (Fig. 1). There is clearly a significant problem in the healing of anastomoses in the large intestines, and this is a subject which has received a great deal of attention in clinical and laboratory studies.

The vast majority of clinical studies have been of a retrospective nature, involving the analysis of case records of patients undergoing anastomosis of the large intestine. With regression-analysis techniques it may be possible to demonstrate that certain clinical variables are associated with anastomotic dehiscence; the significance of these observations, however, is frequently in doubt, and often the case records provide only limited or incomplete information.

The problem of the interpretation of retrospective clinical studies has led to other modes of investigation. Studies of experimental animals permit the examination of specific abnormalities and their effects on colonic healing; and with them tentative conclusions based on retrospective clinical studies can be evaluated. Inevitably, however, the results of animal studies must be interpreted with caution. What happens to colonic anastomoses in rats, rabbits, and other animals may not apply in the human colon, and final proof is required in prospec-

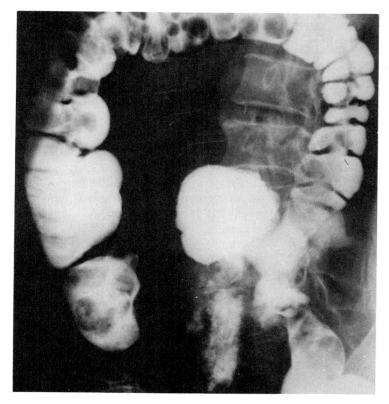

FIG. 1. *Gastrografin enema performed on the fourteenth postoperative day showing a large defect in an anastomoses of the left colon. This leak was not apparent clinically.*

tive clinical studies. Ideally, these studies should be designed as randomized, prospective trials to test the effects of specific prophylaxis or therapy in the management of colonic anastomoses.

In this chapter the results of recent clinical and laboratory studies of the factors affecting colonic healing are described.

FACTORS AFFECTING COLONIC HEALING

Clinical Study

The case records of 203 patients undergoing colonic anastomosis in Leeds were analysed, and it was found that certain clinical variables were associated with anastomotic dehiscence.

Factors Associated with Anastomotic Dehiscence

Age of patient over 60 years
Hypoproteinemia
Advanced malignancy
Surgery for fixed tumors
Inadequate mechanical bowel preparation
Low anterior resection of the rectum

Dehiscence was significantly more common in the elderly and in malnourished patients. There was also a higher incidence of dehiscence in patients with advanced malignant disease (trauma), and this association seemed to be largely related to the high incidence of dehiscence in patients undergoing surgery for fixed tumors. Other factors associated with a significant incidence of anastomotic dehiscence were inadequate mechanical preparation of the bowel and low, anterior resection of the rectum with low pelvic anastomosis.

Trauma and malnutrition, factors which appear to be involved in the pathogenesis of anastomotic dehiscence, have been examined in laboratory studies.

Surgery of Fixed Tumors

It was found that patients who had anastomoses after the removal of fixed tumors of the colon or rectum had a significantly higher incidence of dehiscence compared with those in whom there was no fixation of the bowel (Table 1). There was also a slightly higher incidence of anastomotic dehiscence after operations complicated by inflamma-

Table 1. The Incidence of Anastomotic Dehiscence After Operations
for Fixed Tumors and Operations Complicated by Inflammatory
Adhesion of the Bowel

Fixation of Bowel	No. of Patients	Anastomotic Dehiscence	Incidence of Dehiscence (%)
No fixation	130	11	8
Fixation by tumor	34	11*	32
Fixation by inflammation	39	6	15

Irvin TT, Goligher JC: Br J Surg 60:461, 1973
* Significantly higher incidence of dehiscence compared with no fixation (χ^2 = 11.47, p < 0.001).

tory adhesions of the bowel, but this was not a statistically significant factor in anastomotic dehiscence.

This observation on the surgery of fixed tumors had not been described previously, but other clinical studies have shown that colonic operations complicated by excessive blood loss are associated with a high incidence of anastomotic dehiscence (Whitaker et al. 1970; Schrock et al. 1973). It seemed possible that these different observations might be related and that they may be relevant to some recent observations on the effects of trauma on wound healing. It has been shown that remote trauma has an adverse effect on wound collagen synthesis and tensile strength, probably as a result of hypovolemia and tissue hypoxia (Lundgren and Zederfeldt 1969; Hunt and Pai 1972). There is also evidence that trauma may have important systemic effects on the immunological defense mechanisms and that it may result in an increase susceptibility to bacterial infections (Ollodart and Mansberger 1965; Conolly et al. 1969; Scovill and Saba 1973).

Effect of Trauma on Colonic Healing

The local and systemic effects of trauma on colonic healing were examined in rats. The precise experimental protocol is detailed elsewhere (Irvin and Hunt 1974a). The animals were given end-to-end anastomoses in the left colon, and separate groups of animals were subjected to different types of trauma.

Local Trauma: In this group the surgery of fixed tumors was simulated by producing abdominal trauma in the vicinity of the anastomosis (Fig. 2). A biopsy of muscle was taken from the posterior abdominal wall close to the anastomosis.

Remote Abdominal Trauma: In this group similar abdominal trauma was produced on the opposite side of the abdomen, remote from the anastomosis (Fig. 3).

Extra-abdominal Trauma: In a third group of animals a different type of remote trauma was produced. These animals were subjected to extra-abdominal trauma in the form of a closed fracture of the femur (Fig. 4).

Combined Local and Remote Trauma: In a further group of animals the effects of a combination of local trauma and remote extra-abdominal trauma were studied using the techniques described above (Fig. 5).

Control Group: A fifth group of control animals were given colonic anastomoses, and these animals were not subjected to additional trauma.

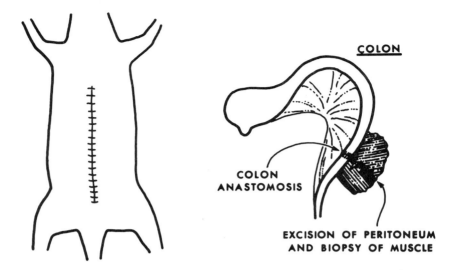

FIG. 2.   Local abdominal trauma: retroperitoneal muscle biopsy was obtained in the vicinity of the anastomosis. (Irvin TT, Hunt TK: Br J Surg 61:430, 1974)

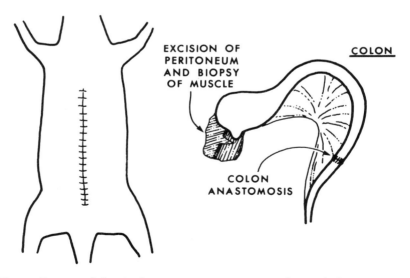

FIG. 3.   Remote abdominal trauma: a retroperitoneal muscle biopsy was obtained on the opposite side of the abdomen, remote from the anastomosis. (Irvin TT, Hunt TK: Br J Surg 61:430, 1974)

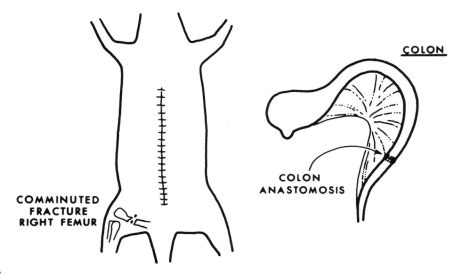

FIG. 4.   Extra-abdominal trauma: a closed comminuted fracture of the femur. (Irvin TT, Hunt TK: Br J Surg 61:430, 1974)

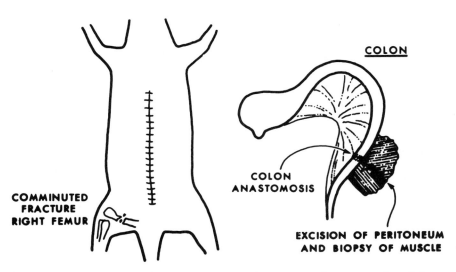

FIG. 5.   Combined trauma: local abdominal trauma and remote extra-abdominal trauma. (Irvin TT, Hunt TK: Br J Surg 61:430, 1974)

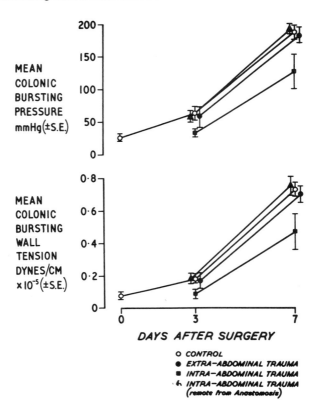

FIG. 6.   Measurements of colonic bursting pressure and bursting wall tension in anastomosis in control and traumatized animals. (Irvin TT, Hunt TK: Br J Surg 61:430, 1974)

The incidence of anastomotic dehiscence in the different groups of animals was recorded, and the effects of the different types of trauma on colonic healing were compared by measurements of the bursting pressure, bursting wall tension, and total collagen content of the anastomoses.

Figure 6 shows the measurements of bursting pressure and bursting wall tension in anastomoses on the third and seventh postoperative days in four groups of rats: the controls, the group given extra-abdominal trauma, the group that received abdominal trauma in the vicinity of the anastomosis, and the group that received trauma remote from the anastomosis. The measurements in the group subjected to local trauma close to the anastomosis were significantly lower than those of control animals, but there was no significant difference between the results of controls and animals which received remote abdominal or extra-abdominal trauma.

Table 2 shows the incidence of anastomotic dehiscence on the seventh postoperative day in the traumatized animals: those which received local trauma close to the anastomosis and those which were subjected to a combination of local trauma and remote extra-abdominal trauma. When the results are compared with those of control animals, it can be seen that there was a significantly higher incidence of dehiscence in traumatized animals. There was no significant difference, however, in the incidence of dehiscence in animals given local trauma alone and those that received a combination of local and remote trauma, although there was a higher mortality in the latter group.

Table 3 shows the collagen concentration in anastomoses on the seventh postoperative day in control animals and animals subjected to local abdominal trauma. The collagen concentration in traumatized animals was lower than that of controls, and it was significantly lower in the disrupted anastomoses of animals subjected to local trauma.

The results show that the local effect of trauma is paramount in the pathogenesis of anastomotic dehiscence. In this study, local trauma occurring close to the colonic anastomosis resulted in a reduced accumulation of wound collagen, diminished colonic tensile strength, and a significant incidence of anastomotic dehiscence.

What is the nature of the local effect of trauma on colon healing? This is a question which we have examined in further studies (Irvin and Hunt 1974b). It was postulated that local trauma results in conditions that favor the development of peritoneal sepsis and that infec-

Table 2. Incidence of Anastomotic Dehiscence in Control Animals, Animals Subjected to Local Abdominal Trauma, and Animals Given a Combination of Local and Remote (Extra-abdominal) Trauma

	No. of Animals	Anastomotic Dehiscence	Incidence of Dehiscence (%)
Control	27	0	0
Local abdominal trauma	27	7*	25.9
Combined local and remote (extra-abdominal) trauma	28	9+	32.1

Irvin TT, Hunt TK: Br J Surg 61:430, 1974
* *Significantly higher incidence of dehiscence compared with the control group ($\chi^2 = 8.04$, $p < 0.01$).*
+ Death resulted from anastomotic dehiscence in 4 animals.

Table 3.   Collagen Concentration in Anastomoses of Control Animals and in the Intact and Disrupted Anastomoses of Animals Subjected to Local Abdominal Trauma

	No. of Animals	Mean Colonic Collagen Concentration (μg/ mg dry tissue ± SEM)
Control	27	113.8 ± 4.14
Trauma		
Intact anastomoses	39	95.8 ± 2.80
Disrupted anastomoses	12	88.0 ± 3.26*

Irvin TT, Hunt TK: Br J Surg 61:430, 1974
* Significant reduction in collagen concentration compared with the control group (t = 3.89, p < 0.001).

tion is the immediate cause of anastomotic failure. This hypothesis was examined in rats using the same trauma model (see Fig. 2), and we deliberately attempted to prevent postoperative peritoneal sepsis in traumatized animals. Two methods were used to prevent peritoneal infection.

Preliminary Defunctioning Colostomy: In one group of animals a preliminary defunctioning colostomy was made four weeks before the animals were subjected to colonic anastomosis and local abdominal trauma (Fig. 7). The presence of a defunctioning colostomy resulted in a marked reduction in the bacterial content of the colon at the time of operation.

Intraperitoneal Antibiotic: In a second group of animals 5 ml of normal saline containing 10 mg of the antibiotic sodium cephalothin was placed in the peritoneal cavity before the abdomen was closed at the end of the colonic operation (Fig. 8). The choice of this antibiotic was based on preliminary studies of the antibiotic sensitivity of the rat fecal flora.

The results of the study are shown in Table 4. The incidence of anastomotic dehiscence on the seventh postoperative day in the two groups of test animals is compared with that in a control group of animals subjected to local abdominal trauma. The presence of a defunctioning colostomy provided significant protection for anastomoses in traumatized animals. There were no dehiscences in colostomy animals. There was also a very low incidence of dehiscence in animals

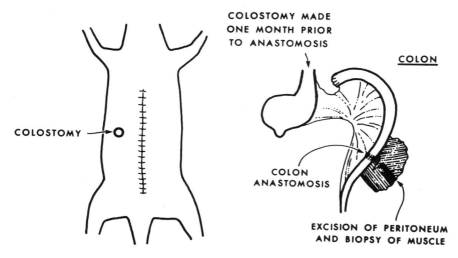

FIG. 7. A defunctioning colostomy was made 4 weeks before subjecting animals to colonic anastomoses and local abdominal trauma. (Irvin TT, Hunt TK: Br J Surg 61:437, 1974)

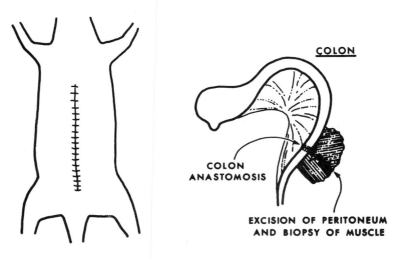

FIG. 8. Sodium cephalothin (10 mg in 5 ml normal saline) was placed in the peritoneal cavity on completion of the anastomosis in traumatized animals. (Irvin TT, Hunt TK: Br J Surg 61:437, 1974)

Table 4.   The Incidence of Anastomotic Dehiscence in Colostomy Animals, Antibiotic-treated Animals, and a Control Group

	No. of Animals	Anastomotic Dehiscence	Incidence of Dehiscence (%)
Control (local abdominal trauma)	27	5	18.5
Intraperitoneal antibiotic	28	1	3.6
Defunctioning colostomy	22	0*	0

Irvin TT, Hunt TK: Br J Surg 61:437, 1974
* Significantly lower incidence of dehiscence compared with the control group $(\chi^2 = 4.54, p < 0.05)$.

given intraperitoneal cephalothin; the numbers of animals are small, however, and the difference between antibiotic-treated animals and controls is not quite statistically significant. It appears, however, that peritoneal infection is the immediate cause of anastomotic dehiscence in traumatized animals.

The results of these laboratory studies may have distinct relevance to the clinical observations that colonic operations involving excessive blood loss or the removal of fixed tumors result in a high incidence of anastomotic dehiscence. It appears that it is the local effect of these operations that affects colonic healing and that local peritoneal infection is the immediate cause of anastomotic dehiscence. Experimental studies have shown that infection has an adverse effect on the healing of colonic anastomoses (Rothenberg et al. 1959; Yamakawa 1971), and it appears that this is the result of a disturbance of colonic collagen metabolism. Hawley (1969) concluded that infection results in increased lysis of mature colonic collagen but recent observations have suggested that the disturbance of collagen metabolism may be more complex. Infection may have an adverse effect on collagen synthesis, and it may cause increased lysis of newly formed colonic collagen (Irvin 1975; also see Chapter 14).

There is now clearly a need for prospective clinical studies of patients undergoing extensive colonic procedures and operations involving the removal of fixed tumors. The results of the experimental studies suggest that the most useful clinical study would be a randomized prospective trial of different types of therapy designed to prevent the development of peritoneal sepsis after such operations.

Malnutrition

Clinical studies have demonstrated that malnutrition and hypoproteinemia are associated with impaired abdominal wound healing (Localio et al. 1948), and there seems to be an association between malnutrition and the dehiscence of colonic anastomoses (Irvin and Goligher 1973). In the retrospective clinical study in Leeds it was found that patients who developed dehiscence of colonic anastomoses had significantly lower plasma proteins than those who avoided this complication Table 5).

Studies of experimental animals have confirmed that malnutrition and protein deprivation have adverse effects on wound healing. Many of these studies have suggested that the relationship may be extremely sensitive, and it has been shown that minor degrees of malnutrition adversely affect the healing of skin wounds (Williamson et al. 1951; Udupa et al. 1956; Rosenberg and Caldwell 1965). There is less information regarding colon healing, but Daly and his colleagues (1972) studied the healing of colonic anastomoses in protein-starved rats and claimed that colonic healing was affected within one week of protein deprivation, when the average loss of body weight amounted to only 2 percent. The same group (Daly et al. 1974) claimed that colonic healing in normal rats was impaired by minor degrees of dietary deprivation during the postoperative period and that these changes could be prevented by postoperative intravenous hyperalimentation.

The possible therapeutic implications of these experimental studies are considerable, but it should be noted that the studies were limited to measurements of colonic bursting pressure in protein-starved animals and that there have been no detailed biochemical studies of the effects of malnutrition on the colon.

Some recent studies of the effects of malnutrition on the colon have

Table 5. Plasma Protein Measurements in Patients With and Without Dehiscence of Colonic Anastomoses (mean g/100 ml $\pm$ SD)

	Total Protein*	Albumin†
No dehiscence (n = 89)	7.2 $\pm$ 0.86	3.9 $\pm$ 0.52
Dehiscence (n = 17)	6.6 $\pm$ 0.53	3.4 $\pm$ 0.71

Irvin TT, Goligher JC: Br J Surg 60:461, 1973
* $p < 0.01$; † $p < 0.001$.

Table 6.   Constituents of Protein-free and Normal Rat Diets
(% of total by weight)

Dietary Constituents	Control (Normal) Diet	Protein-Free Diet
Casein	25	—
Cornstarch	60	85
Hydrogenated cottonseed oil	8	8
Hawk-Oser salt mixture	4	4
Vitamin supplement	1	1
Cellulose non-nutritive fiber	2	2

Irvin TT, Hunt TK: Ann Surg 180:765, 1974

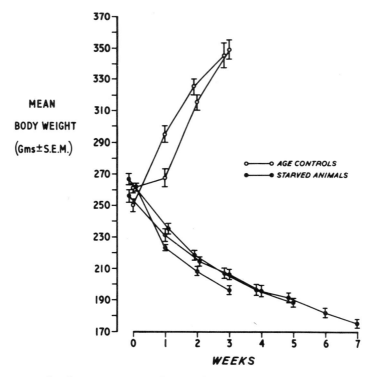

FIG. 9.   Weight changes in control animals (age controls) and animals starved of protein for 3, 5, and 7 weeks. (Irvin TT, Hunt TK: Ann Surg 180:765, 1974)

revealed a rather different pattern of colonic healing (Irvin and Hunt 1974c). The studies were made in young adult rats deprived of protein for periods of 3, 5, and 7 weeks; test animals were compared with controls fed a normal diet. The protein-free and normal rat diets were based on the recommendations of Hegstead and Chang (1965) (Table 6). The effects of malnutrition on the uninjured colon and on the healing of end-to-end colonic anastomoses were studied, using measurements of colonic bursting pressure, colonic bursting wall tension, and the collagen content of anastomoses.

Control animals gained weight on the normal diet but there was a progressive loss of weight in protein-starved animals, and this amounted to a 34 percent reduction after 7 weeks (Fig. 9). There was thus a significant difference in the size of control and protein-starved animals (Fig. 10), and the colon of test and control animals was of different

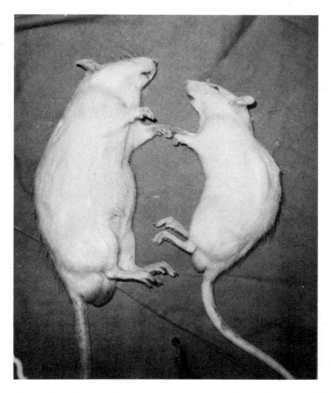

FIG. 10. *Control and protein-starved animals of similar age. The protein-starved animal (on the right) is markedly smaller than the control.*

size (Fig. 11). A greater degree of technical difficulty was encountered in making anastomoses in the smaller colon of protein-starved animals, and we felt that this difference between test and control animals introduced problems in the interpretation of results. For this reason two further groups of control animals were studied. These were younger animals of similar size and weight to the protein-starved animals, and the size of the colon in these control animals was equivalent to that of test animals. There were thus three groups of control animals: a group of similar age (age controls) and two groups of younger animals (weight controls) of similar size and weight to the protein-starved animals.

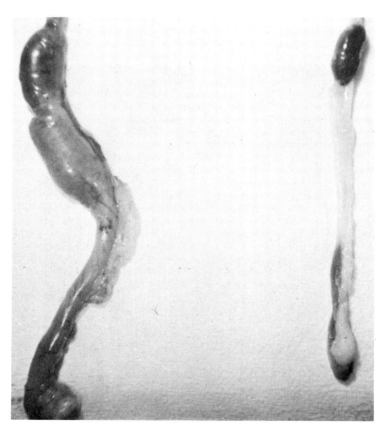

FIG. 11. *The colon of the protein-starved animal (right) is of much smaller caliber than that of a control animal of similar age (left).*

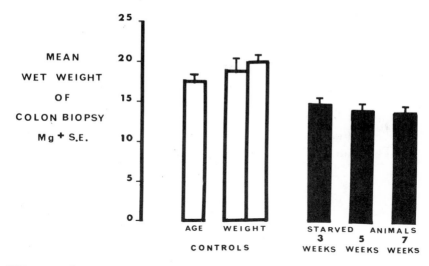

FIG. 12. *The wet weight of standard biopsies of the uninjured colon of age controls, the two groups of weight controls, and animals deprived of protein for 3, 5, and 7 weeks.*

CHANGES IN THE UNINJURED COLON. Figure 12 shows the wet weight of standard colon biopsies obtained from the uninjured colon of age controls, the two groups of weight controls, and groups of test animals deprived of protein for 3, 5, and 7 weeks. The wet weight of the colon in protein-starved animals was significantly lower than that of control animals.

Figure 13 shows the total collagen content of the colon biopsies and measurements of the colonic collagen concentration. The concentration of collagen in the colon of protein-starved animals was significantly higher than that of control animals, resulting from the removal of noncollagenous components of colonic tissue in response to protein deprivation. Collagen was not removed from the colon to a significant extent until protein deprivation had lasted seven weeks. There was a significant difference in the collagen content of the colon in age controls and weight controls, but these age-related changes in tissue collagen appear to be a normal physiological feature in rodents (Zika and Klein 1971).

COLONIC ANASTOMOSES. Figure 14 shows measurements of colonic bursting pressure and colonic bursting wall tension on the third and seventh postoperative days in anastomoses in age controls and groups

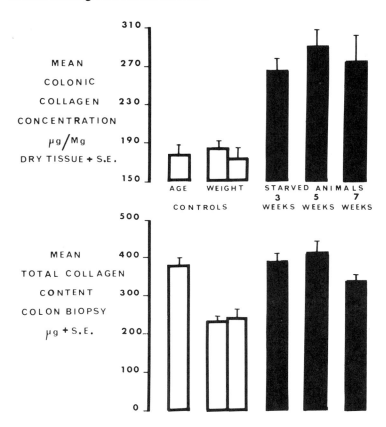

FIG. 13.   *The collagen content of colon biopsies and measurements of colonic collagen concentration in age controls, the two groups of weight controls, and test animals starved for 3, 5, and 7 weeks.*

of test animals starved of protein for 3, 5, and 7 weeks. Significant decreases were found in the group starved for 7 weeks.

The total collagen content of the anastomoses in the same groups of animals are shown in Figure 15, and it can be seen that the collagen content of anastomoses in the group deprived of protein for seven weeks was significantly lower than that of control animals.

Figure 16 shows the total collagen content of anastomoses on the day of surgery and on the third and seventh postoperative days in age controls, the two groups of weight controls, and a group of test animals starved for 7 weeks. The normal pattern of colon healing is shown in the group of age controls. There was a slight reduction in the collagen content of anastomoses on the third postoperative day, but thereafter there was a phase of collagen synthesis and a marked increase in the collagen content of anastomoses. The collagen content of anastomoses in weight controls and protein-starved animals on the day of surgery was significantly lower than the value in age controls, and this is a reflection of the pre-existing differences in the collagen content of the uninjured colon in test animals and control animals of differing age. Similar differences were apparent on the third postoperative day, but after the third day there was evidence of rapid collagen synthesis in all control animals. There was very little evidence of collagen synthesis in protein-starved animals, however, and the collagen content of anastomoses in starved animals on the seventh postoperative day was significantly lower than the values in the three groups of control animals.

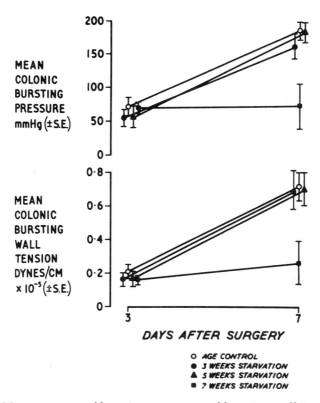

FIG. 14. Measurements of bursting pressure and bursting wall tension in anastomoses in age controls, and test animals starved for 3, 5, and 7 weeks. (Irvin TT, Hunt TK: Ann Surg 180:765, 1974)

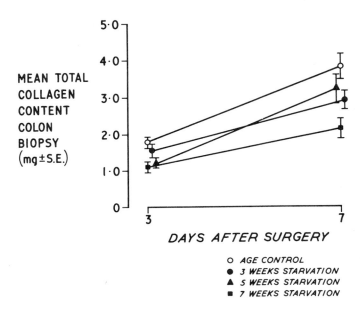

FIG. 15. The collagen content of anastomoses in age controls, and test animals starved for 3, 5, and 7 weeks. (Irvin TT, Hunt TK: Ann Surg 180:765, 1974)

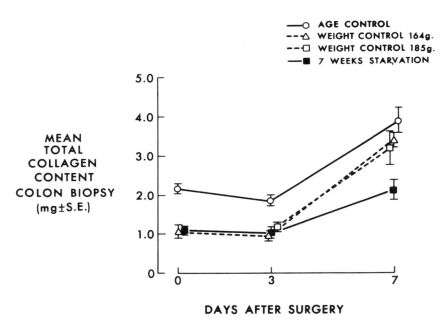

FIG. 16. The collagen content of anastomoses in age controls, weight controls, and a group of test animals starved of protein for 7 weeks. (Irvin TT, Hunt TK: Ann Surg 180:765, 1974)

Figure 17 shows the collagen concentration in anastomoses on the third and seventh postoperative days in age controls and the groups of test animals starved of protein for 3, 5, and 7 weeks. In protein-starved animals, the collagen concentration in dry colonic tissue was slightly higher than that of age controls on the third day, and this is a reflection of the pre-existing differences in the collagen concentration in the uninjured colon of test and control animals. There was a slight increase in the concentration of collagen in dry colonic tissue between the third and seventh days. The results in wet colonic tissue show a similar trend, except that there is a striking difference in the behavior of anastomoses in animals starved for 7 weeks. In this group there was a significant reduction in the collagen concentration in wet colonic

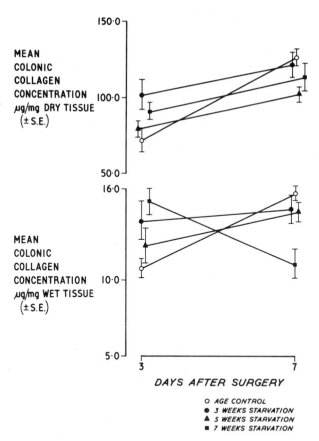

FIG. 17. Measurements of the collagen concentration in dry and wet colonic tissue in anastomoses in age controls and groups of test animals starved for 3, 5, and 7 weeks. (Irvin TT, Hunt TK: Ann Surg 180:765, 1974)

tissue between the third and seventh days, and these results indicate that edema was a feature of wound healing.

The results of this study indicate that the healing of colonic anatomoses was affected only in animals starved of protein for 7 weeks. These animals lost 34 percent of their body weight, and colonic collagen synthesis and the tensile strength of colonic anastomoses were significantly inferior to the values in control animals. The study does not support the conclusions from previous studies that minor degrees of malnutrition have important effects on colonic healing, and there appears to be no rational basis for the *routine* use of postoperative intravenous hyperalimentation for patients undergoing colon excisions.

CONCLUSIONS

Multiple factors are involved in the pathogenesis of anastomotic dehiscence. Several factors which may be implicated have been identified in retrospective clinical studies, and studies of animal models have helped to evaluate their precise effect on colonic healing.

The two experimental studies described in this chapter have defined the effects of abdominal trauma and malnutrition on colonic healing but further studies of these and other factors are required. We will of necessity continue to operate on malnourished patients. For those patients who require extensive colonic operations, we must develop techniques which will reduce the incidence of anastomotic dehiscence. Further experimental studies may be required; but, finally, the effects of specific prophylaxis or therapy must be examined in randomized prospective clinical trials. Such studies have already shown the significance of mechanical bowel preparation and suture techniques in colon surgery (Goligher et al. 1970; Rosenberg et al. 1971; Irvin et al. 1973; Everett 1975).

REFERENCES

Conolly WB, Hunt TK, Sonne M, Dunphy JE: Influence of distant trauma on local wound infection. Surg Gynecol Obstet 128:173, 1969

Daly JM, Steiger E, Vars HM, Dudrick SJ: Postoperative oral and intravenous nutrition. Ann Surg 180:709, 1974

Daly JM, Vars HM, Dudrick SJ: Effects of protein depletion on strength of colonic anastomoses. Surg Gynecol Obstet 134:15, 1972

Everett WG: A comparison of one layer and two layer techniques for colorectal anastomosis. Br J Surg 62:135, 1975

Goligher JC, Morris C, McAdam WAF, DeDombal FT, Johnston D: A controlled trial of inverting versus everting intestinal suture in clinical large bowel surgery. Br J Surg 57:817, 1970

Hawley PR: The aetiology of colonic anastomotic leaks with special reference to the role of collagenase. M.S. thesis, University of London, 1969

Hegstead DM, Chang Y: Protein utilization in growing rats. J Nutr 85:159, 1965

Hunt TK, Pai MP: The effect of varying ambient oxygen tensions on wound metabolism and collagen synthesis. Surg Gynecol Obstet 135:561, 1972

Irvin TT: Collagen metabolism in infected colonic anastomoses. Br J Surg 62:659, 1975

Irvin TT, Goligher JC: Aetiology of disruption of intestinal anastomoses. Br J Surg 60:461, 1973

Irvin TT, Goligher JC, Johnston D: A randomised prospective clinical trial of single-layer and two-layer inverting intestinal anastomoses. Br J Surg 60:457, 1973

Irvin TT, Hunt TK: The effect of trauma on colonic healing. Br J Surg 61:430, 1974a

Irvin TT, Hunt TK: Pathogenesis and prevention of disruption of colonic anastomoses in traumatized rats. Br J Surg 61:437, 1974b

Irvin TT, Hunt TK: Effect of malnutrition on colonic healing. Ann Surg 180:765, 1974c

Localio SA, Chassin JL, Hinton JW: Tissue protein depletion. A factor in wound disruption. Surg Gynecol Obstet 86:107, 1948

Lundgren CEG, Zederfeldt B: Influence of low oxygen pressure on wound healing. Acta Chir Scand 135:555, 1969

Ollodart R, Mansberger AR: The effect of hypovolemic shock on bacterial defense. A J Surg 110:302, 1965

Rosenberg F, Caldwell FT: Effect of single amino acid supplementation upon the rate of wound contraction and wound morphology in protein depleted rats. Surg Gynecol Obstet 121:1021, 1965

Rosenberg IL, Graham NG, DeDombal FT, Goligher JC: Preparation of the intestine in patients undergoing major large bowel surgery, mainly for neoplasms of the colon and rectum. Br J Surg 58:266, 1971

Rothenberg H, Chassin J, Scher S, Treitler B, Lear PE: Bowel anastomosis in the presence of peritonitis. Surg Forum 10:201, 1959

Schrock TR, Deveney CW, Dunphy JE: Factors contributing to leakage of colonic anastomoses. Ann Surg 177:513, 1973

Scovill WA, Saba TM: Humoral recognition deficiency in the aetiology of reticulo endothelial depression induced by surgery. Ann Surg 178:59, 1973

Udupa KN, Woessner JF, Dunphy JE: The effect of methionine on the production of mucopolysaccharides and collagen in healing wounds of protein-depleted animals. Surg Gynecol Obstet 102:639, 1956

Whitaker BL, Dixon RA, Greatorex G: Anastomotic failure in relation to blood transfusion and blood loss. Proc R Soc Med 63:751, 1970

Williamson MB, McCarthy TH, Fromm HJ: Relation of protein nutrition to the healing of experimental wounds. Proc Soc Exp Biol Med 77:302, 1951

Yamakawa T, Patin CS, Sobel S, Morgenstern L: Healing of colonic anastomoses following resection for experimental "diverticulitis." Arch Surg 103:17, 1971

Zika Jocelyn M, Klein L: Relative and absolute changes in skin collagen mass in the rat. Biochim Biophys Acta 229:509, 1971

Comment

This study is the scientific apex of this field of investigation. Mr. Irvin's passionate pursuit of perfection has led him to the most exacting studies yet done on the development of anastomotic integrity in the colon. Its results differ somewhat from what I originally expected. His excellent work, therefore, arouses certain questions in my mind. For example, other investigators have long since proved that remote trauma of the degree he used has a deleterious effect on repair and resistance to infection in skin and subcutaneous wounds. It is not clear to me why this effect is not detectable in the colonic anastomosis. Perhaps circulating catecholamines affect colonic circulation less than skin circulation, or perhaps sympathetic nervous supply differs.

In any case, however, Mr. Irvin has clearly shown that one of the paramount enemies of colonic repair is local trauma. Among other things, he has shown the value of a functionally intact peritoneum. This study should be remembered by every trauma surgeon—not just as an admonition that repair or reanastomosis of colon wounds may be hazardous, but because it allows the surgeon to judge those occasions in which a simple closure is possible—that is, in small knife wounds treated with antibiotics shortly after injury, in which the local trauma is slight and, we might add, in which there are no other significant injuries or shock, since the patient must always heal the body-wall wound without infection.

Mr. Irvin has probably solved a common surgical paradox. Most experienced surgeons have left the operating table with the feeling that they have done the perfect technical anastomosis only to encounter a leak sometime later. When they reoperate, they may find that the leak is not in the anastomosis at all but, instead, is a few millimeters or a centimeter proximal. Mr. Irvin has shown in a simple and convincing way that, at least in some cases, the infection precedes and probably causes the leak. He has made a powerful case for preventive antibiotics or antiseptics in colon surgery and just as convincingly a case for clean, gentle, technical operations.

Mr. Irvin did not essay to discuss the effect of infection on colon synthesis in wounds although he alludes to it with regard to his own results. In this study, he finds collagen *accumulation* unequivocally depressed by infection. In studies of skin repair, others have shown a similar effect, but still others have found *increased* collagen accumulation as a result of infection. Several possibilities seem to resolve this conflict, and all are probably operative to one degree or another in varying circumstances. The first is that the pattern of collagen deposition and cross-linking may change under the effect of infections. The wall of an abscess is thick and collagenous, but its center is free of collagen and filled with white cells and bacteria. Second, the peritonitis he produced by trauma and contamination may decrease collagen synthesis through a systemic effect, one of the mediators possibly being hypovolemia, which often follows peritonitis. Third, different infecting organisms may have differing effects on collagen metabolism. For instance, it seems to me through clinical experience that anaerobic infections seem to paralyze collagen synthesis while some aerobic infections (and some have been tested) seem to stimulate it. Perhaps the reasons for this stimulation lie in Dr. Ross's observations (Chapter 1) on the effect of stimulating macrophages. At any rate, the important conclusion is obvious in Mr. Irvin's study: Whether or not more collagen is formed, the strength of the anastomosis is jeopardized by infection.

Determinants of the Unsuccessful Colonic Anastomosis in Humans

14

Theodore R. Schrock

The unsuccessful anastomosis was an important problem at the inception of colonic surgery,[1] and it remains a major concern today. In one recent study, anastomotic failure caused one-third of the deaths and much of the morbidity from operations on the large bowel.[2]

In the early part of this century, surgeons departed from the view that primary anastomosis of the colon was absolutely unsafe and evolved the concept that anastomosis was permissible if rigid criteria were met.[1,3] Armed with antibiotics and other advances, the modern surgeon believes that, except in certain situations, primary anastomosis is much preferred over staged procedures. Clinical experience and experiments in animals have defined some of the mechanisms by which healing is impaired, and the present review will summarize current knowledge of determinants of anastomotic failure in humans.

Studies of colonic anastomoses in humans are limited by the difficulty of ascertaining whether an anastomosis has healed or leaked. Two approaches to the problems are available: retrospective and prospective. Table 1 shows the incidence of dehiscence of colorectal anastomoses studied retrospectively in one institution[2] and prospectively in another.[4] In the retrospective study, medical records were reviewed for evidence of anastomotic failure: fistula, peritonitis, or unexplained sepsis. In the prospective study, digital rectal, sigmoidoscopic, and radiographic contrast examinations were obtained routinely in the postoperative period. Dehiscence was detected in an additional 36 percent of patients by this careful search, and the overall incidence of leakage rose to 51 percent. The diagnostic manipulations probably did not cause breaks in intact anastomoses in view of the interval after

Table 1.   Rates of Anastomotic Dehiscence Determined Retrospectively
or Prospectively

Anastomotic Dehiscence	Retrospective* (n = 368)	Prospective† (n = 73)
Clinically apparent	34 (9.2%)	11 (15%)
Special studies	—	26 (36%)
Total	34 (9.2%)	37 (51%)

*From Schrock TR, et al: Ann Surg 177:513, 1973
†From Goligher JC, et al: Br J Surg 57:109, 1970

operation and the care exercised. Although the prospective method reveals the true incidence of anastomotic leak, many of the dehiscences were subclinical, did not prolong recovery, and could not be considered "failures." Retrospective studies overlook the subclinical leaks and detect only the major, clinically significant dehiscences.

The determinants of the unsuccessful colonic anastomosis in humans may be grouped into three categories: technical, local, and systemic.

TECHNICAL DETERMINANTS

Technical Errors

Excellent blood supply is a requisite for anastomotic healing, and blood supply can be impaired by a variety of technical errors: ligation of critical mesenteric vessels, hematoma formation at the suture line, sutures tied too tightly, tension on the anastomosis due to failure to mobilize the colon adequately, and trauma to the tissues by instruments or rough handling.

Details of suture technique vary among surgeons; neither single nor two-layer anastomosis has been proved superior to the other.[5] Again, the effect of gentleness and care probably outweighs that of specific suture techniques. Sutures must be placed carefully to avoid gaps in the anastomosis, and tissue must not be inverted excessively. Halsted demonstrated that excessively inverted tissue compromised the lumen and became ischemic, thus promoting infection in the bowel wall.[6] Everting technique was condemned in a prospective, controlled trial, which showed that overt fecal fistula occurred in 43 percent of everting anastomoses compared with 8.6 percent of inverting anastomoses.[7]

Drains

Some surgeons believe that rubber or plastic drains facilitate healing by prevention of blood, serum, or purulent collections near the anastomosis. It was shown years ago that drains in animals are rapidly sealed off from the peritoneal cavity,[8] and more recent studies suggest that drainage of colonic anastomoses is both ineffective and harmful.[9,10] Drains are foreign bodies which promote sepsis, interfere with vital peritoneal defense mechanisms, and prevent the sealing of small leaks by adjacent omentum or bowel.[10] There is no scientific support for the use of drains in intraperitoneal anastomoses of the large bowel.[9,11]

The low rectal anastomosis may be an exception, however, because it lies outside the peritoneal cavity. Leakage in this area results in part from the collection of infected material behind the rectum and rupture into the lumen, usually through the posterior midline of the anastomosis.[12,13] Controlled studies are lacking here too, but most surgeons employ some form of drainage of low rectal anastomoses.[11] Drains are detrimental in any location if they lie in direct contact with the suture line.

Proximal Diversion

Proximal decompression or diversion by means of cecostomy or colostomy has been advocated to promote anastomotic healing. Table 2 shows the incidence of leakage and the mortality rates in patients who had leakage from colorectal anastomoses with or without proximal decompression. In this study and in others like it, surgeons preferred not to add proximal decompression unless they were concerned about the security of the anastomosis. The data confirm previous reports that leakage can occur despite proximal decompression, but if an anastomosis dehisces the mortality rate is much lower in the presence of fecal diversion.[14-19] Cecostomy is less effective than colostomy in blunting the consequences of anastomotic failure.[14,16,19]

Table 2. Effects of Proximal Colostomy or Cecostomy on Leakage Rate and Mortality of Leakage from Colorectal Anastomoses

	Anastomoses	Leaks	Mortality of Leaks
Colostomy or cecostomy	129	15 (11.6%)	13.3%
No colostomy or cecostomy	238	19 (8.0%)	35.3%

From Schrock TR, et al: Ann Surg 177:513, 1973

Table 3.   Anastomotic Leakage Rates in Various
Segments of Colon

Segments Anastomosed	Anastomoses	Leaks
Small bowel to right colon	577	22 (3.8%)
Left colon to left colon	408	13 (3.2%)
Left colon to rectum	368	34 (9.2%)

From Schrock TR, et al: Ann Surg 177:513, 1973

LOCAL DETERMINANTS

The segment of colon that is anastomosed, abnormal bowel, intralumical pressure, and infection are local determinants of anastomotic healing.

Segment of Colon

Table 3 shows the leakage rates from anastomoses in different parts of the large bowel after resection for various diseases. Rectal anastomoses failed more often than others, but the data do not support the contention that primary anastomosis of small bowel to right colon is safer than left colocolic anastomosis.

Surgeons were more willing to anastomose primarily on the right in emergencies in this series, but if the cases were analyzed further to exclude those patients with infection at the time of operation, the leakage rate was still as high in the right colon as in the left colon (Table 4). Abuse of primary anastomosis on the right side in emergency situations resulted in prohibitively high mortality in one series.[20]

Table 4.   Failure Rates of Anastomoses
in the Presence of Infection

Segments Anastomosed	No Infection at Operation		Infection at Operation	
	Anastomoses	Leaks	Anastomoses	Leaks
Small bowel to right colon	422	13 (3.1%)	87	6 (6.9%)
Left colon to left colon	487	12 (2.4%)	58	7 (12.1%)
Colon to rectum	329	26 (7.9%)	39	8 (20.5%)

From Schrock TR, et al: Ann Surg 177:513, 1973

Abnormal Bowel

Inflamed[14,21] or distended[15] colon is hazardous to anastomose. Irradiated colon is notoriously prone to anastomotic dehiscence; the leakage rate was as high as 50 percent after resection of irradiated colon in one study.[22] There is some evidence also that malignant cells at the anastomotic site predispose to leakage.[27]

Intraluminal Pressure

High intraluminal pressure due to distal obstruction is detrimental to anastomotic healing. Contraction of colonic musculature after administration of neostigmine to reverse muscle relaxants has been implicated as a cause of dehiscence,[23] but the relationship has not been proved.

Infection

Infection is a powerful determinant of unsuccessful anastomosis.[2,3,4,17,20,21,24] Table 4 lists the outcome of anastomoses performed in various parts of the large bowel in the presence or absence of abdominal infection (abscess or peritonitis) at the time of operation. Leakage was more frequent in the infected patients regardless of which segment of bowel was used.

If infection is absent at the time the anastomosis is constructed, it may develop postoperatively in patients with inadequately prepared bowel.[3,4,17] In one study, unprepared colon was anastomosed primarily after resection for diverticular disease in 15 patients who had neither abscess nor peritonitis at the time.[27] Two of these patients (13.3 percent) suffered anastomotic dehiscence, probably related to the development of sepsis in or near the anastomosis after operation; this incidence of leakage was similar to that found in patients who had infection already established at operation.

Two local determinants that promote infection, and thus anastomotic failure, are local tissue trauma and blood in the vicinity of the anastomosis.[2,17,25,26,27] Both factors are difficult to assess in the clinical setting, but the duration of the operation and the number of blood transfusions required are crude measures of difficult, traumatic, and bloody dissection; anastomotic dehiscence rates correlated with these parameters in one retrospective study.[27]

Infection is one important reason for the frequent failure of low (extraperitoneal) rectal anastomoses. The inevitable bacterial contamination which is readily disposed of in the peritoneal cavity is not as easily disposed of in the pelvis and produces infection which disrupts the suture line.[12,13] Another sort of evidence that extraperitoneal anastomoses heal poorly is available also. In a series of 19 patients with traumatic perforations of the colon which were managed by suture and exteriorization of that segment of the colon, 11 patients (58 percent) dehisced the exteriorized suture line.[27] Serositis developed on the exposed bowel after a few days, and this type of infection undoubtedly contributed to the loss of anastomotic integrity.

SYSTEMIC DETERMINANTS

Advanced Age

There is a greater likelihood of anastomotic dehiscence in the elderly.[2,17] Leakage occurred in 3.4 percent of patients under 60 years of age compared with 9.6 percent of patients 80 years or older.[27] Several factors are responsible, including slower healing, poorer blood supply, and lowered resistance to infection.

Impaired Delivery of Oxygen

Synthesis of collagen and resistance to infection depend upon adequate supplies of oxygen.[24] Delivery of oxygen can be impaired by systemic factors in addition to actual ligation of mesenteric vessels or errors in suture technique. Extensive remote trauma, hypovolemia, hypotension, or hypoxemia from any cause reduce oxygen delivery, and these factors are associated with a greater likelihood of anastomotic dehiscence.[2,24,25,27] Anastomoses leaked in 31.8 percent of patients who underwent operation for acute massive hemorrhage from the colon; inadequate supply of oxygen was one of several deleterious influences in these cases.[27] Simple anemia did not increase the risk of anastomotic failure. [This is consistent with what is known of anemia and oxygen delivery to wounds—Ed.]

Malnutrition

Experiments in animals show that severe malnutrition adversely affects colonic healing,[28] but quantitative data on this point are difficult to obtain in humans[27] (see Chapter 13).

Systemic Steroids

Animal studies show that the systemic administration of exogenous adrenal corticosteroids interferes with the synthesis of collagen and promotes infection,[24] and many clinical surgeons are convinced that patients receiving corticosteroids have a greater risk of anastomotic failure. One study directed to this question did not confirm this clinical impression,[29] and the influence of corticosteroid administration on colonic healing in patients has not been established.[27]

Other Systemic Determinants

Cancer-chemotherapeutic agents almost certainly impair colonic healing.[24] Associated diseases such as obesity, diabetes mellitus, and renal failure may also be important.[21]

SUMMARY

Numerous technical, local, and systemic factors interact to determine the success of anastomotic healing in the large bowel. Healing is uneventful in most patients, but the balance may be tilted toward leakage by a single powerful determinant, such as infection or ischemia, or by an accumulation of relatively minor determinants. Although there is no substitute for technical excellence in the construction of an anastomosis, surgical judgment—the decision whether to anastomose primarily or not—is also crucial. By weighing the determinants in a clinical situation and deferring anastomosis if necessary, surgeons should be able to lower the incidence of major anastomotic disruption to 2 percent or less.[27]

REFERENCES

1. Dunphy JE: The cut gut. Am J Surg 119:1, 1970
2. Schrock TR, Deveney CW, Dunphy JE: Factors contributing to leakage of colonic anastomoses. Ann Surg 177:513, 1973
3. Dunphy JE: Preoperative preparation of the colon and other factors affecting anastomotic healing. Cancer 28:181, 1971
4. Goligher JC, Graham NG, DeDombal FT: Anastomotic dehiscence after anterior resection of rectum and sigmoid. Br J Surg 57:109, 1970
5. Irvin TT, Goligher JC, Johnston D: A randomized prospective clinical trial of single-layer and two-layer inverting intestinal anastomoses. Br J Surg 60:457, 1973
6. Halsted WS: Circular suture of the intestine—an experimental study. Am J Med Sci 94:436, 1887
7. Goligher JC, Morris C, McAdam WAF, DeDombal FT, Johnston D: A controlled trial of inverting versus everting intestinal suture in clinical large bowel surgery. Br J Surg 57:817, 1970
8. Yates JL: An experimental study of the local effects of peritoneal drainage. Surg Gynecol Obstet 1:473, 1905

9. Berliner SD, Burson LC, Lear PE: Intraperitoneal drains in surgery of the colon. Clinical evaluation of 454 cases. Am J Surg 113:646, 1967
10. Crowson WN, Wilson CS: An experimental study of the effects of drains on colon anastomoses. Am Surg 39:597, 1973
11. Duthie HL: Curent concepts. Drainage of the abdomen. N Engl J Med 287:1081, 1972
12. Collins CD, Talbot CH: Pelvic drainage after anterior resection of the rectum. Arch Surg 99:391, 1969
13. Schaupp WC: Drainge of low anterior anastomoses. Am J Surg 118:627, 1969
14. Botsford TW, Zollinger RM Jr: Diverticulitis of the colon. Surg Gynecol Obstet 128:1209, 1969
15. Colcock BP: Surgical treatment of diverticulitis. Twenty years' experience. Am J Surg 115:264, 1968
16. Garnjobst W, Hardwick C: Further criteria for anastomosis in diverticulitis of the sigmoid colon. Am J Surg 120:264, 1970
17. Irvin TT, Goligher JC: Aetiology of disruption of intestinal anastomoses. Br J Surg 60:461, 1973
18. Miller DW Jr, Wichern WA Jr: Perforated sigmoid diverticulitis. Appraisal of primary versus delayed resection. Am J Surg 121:536, 1971
19. Smithwick RH: Surgical treatment of diverticulitis of the sigmoid. Am J Surg 99: 192, 1960
20. Debas HT, Thomson FB: A critical review of colectomy with anastomosis. Surg Gynecol Obstet 135:747, 1972
21. Morgenstern L, Yamakawa T, Ben-Shoshan M, Lippman H: Anastomotic leakage after low colonic anastomosis. Clinical and experimental aspects. Am J Surg 123:104, 1972
22. Deveney CW, Lewis FR Jr, Schrock TR: Surgical management of radiation injury of the small and large intestine. Dis Colon Rectum 19:25, 1976
23. Bell CMA, Lewis CB: Effect of neostigmine on integrity of ileorectal anastomoses. Br Med J 5618:587, 1968
24. Hunt TK, Hawley PR: Surgical judgment and colonic anastomoses. Dis Colon Rectum 12:167, 3969
25. Irvin TT, Hunt TK: The effect of trauma on colonic healing. Br J Surg 61:430, 1974
26. Irvin TT, Hunt TK: Pathogenesis and prevention of disruption of colonic anastomosis in traumatized rats. Br J Surg 61:437, 1974
27. Schrock TR, Christensen N: Management of perforating injuries of the colon. Surg Gynecol Obstet 135:65, 1972
28. Irvin TT, Hunt TK: Effect of malnutrition on colonic healing. Ann Surg 180:765, 1974
29. Price LA: The effect of systemic steroids on ileorectal anastomosis in ulcerative colitis. Br J Surg 55:839, 1968

Comment

After a chapter on the physiology and pathophysiology of colon repair, mostly as determined in animals, this study economically summarizes the data as determined in humans. Dr. Schrock has assembled the two largest retrospective examinations of colon anastomoses, and much of the data herein reflect the experience of our 2000 cases. He has examined many clinical correlates of unsuccessful outcomes. It is immediately obvious that anastomotic leak in patients can easily be attributed to or correlated with various significant clinical events, but mechanisms cannot easily be determined in clinical studies. For instance, Dr. Schrock points out the association of anastomotic leak with use of blood during operation, and Mr. Irvin elucidates the mechanisms.

I keep the following chart in my mind during all colon operations. I wish we could assign a number to each detrimental factor and forgo primary anastomosis when ˙a critical sum is reached. Unfortunately, we cannot weigh each factor that accurately.

Indications for Staging or Proximal Diversion

Difficult operation with severe associated trauma and blood loss	+ +
Established local infection	+ +
Advanced age	+ +
Radiation with visible tissue change months or years before	
Protein depletion—20 percent weight loss (can be negated with preoperative hyperalimentation)	+
Pelvic anastomosis	+
Current cancer chemotherapy	+
Emergency operation	+
Radiation (curative doses 6 weeks prior)	+
Diabetes	Mild 0, moderate +, severe + +

Uremia	Variable with degree
Continuing steroid therapy with Cushing's syndrome	+
Continuing steroid therapy without Cushing's syndrome	±

Dr. Schrock has stated that steroids have not been demonstrated to be harmful to the colonic anastomosis. Unfortunately, good clinical evidence is hard to find; and he is right that negative evidence has not been assembled. Steroids, however, have demonstrated their deleterious effects on repair so often that, until good positive evidence that they are definitely harmless in the colon is found, I will continue to assume they add to the risk of anastomotic complications.*

---

*As we go to press, Dr. Zederfeldt has told me that recent studies in his laboratory confirm that colon repair is little affected in animals treated with steroids.

Sutures and Wound Repair
15

James C. Forrester

Connective tissue formation proceeds best in the undisturbed wound; this usually means that some form of suture support is required. The key to successful suturing lies in a clear concept both of the wound's individuality as a repair organ and of the physical and biologic characteristics of the suture materials.

THE WOUND

The repair organ is the granulation tissue that fills the wound. This delicate system of cells and capillaries has the general function of connective tissue formation. The fibroblast is the key cell, synthesizing both collagen and intercellular ground substance. Fibroblast activity is critically dependent on a ready supply of oxygen, and it cannot function effectively more than about 50 μ ahead of the nearest normally perfused capillary.[1,2,3] The same rules apply to some of the other tissue cells and the polymorphonuclear cell is particularly vulnerable.[4] In practical terms, the wound must be handled with the utmost gentleness to minimize cell damage and insure good wound perfusion and oxygenation.[5,6,7]

Although collagen is rapidly synthesized by the wound, strength is recovered quite slowly.[8] This has particular relevance to healing in tissues of great natural strength, such as tendon or aponeurosis (Fig. 1). It takes almost three months for aponeurosis to recover 60 percent of its strength. Although there is further recovery by the end of a year, some defect appears to be permanent.

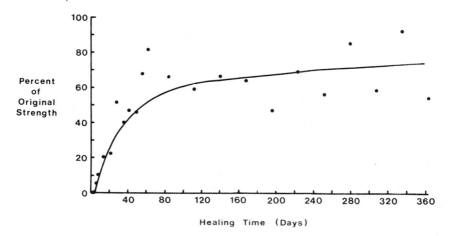

FIG. 1. *Breaking strength of healing aponeurotic wounds. Strength increases rapidly for several weeks but then slows. There is only 70 percent recovery by the end of a year. (After Douglas DM: Br J Surg 40:79, 1952)*

When an incision is closed, marked biochemical changes can be observed in the normal tissues on either side.[9] As far as sutures are concerned, the most important is the active collagenolysis that causes it to soften in the first few postoperative days (Fig. 2). This lytic process is enhanced if the wound becomes infected. If sutures are to hold securely, they should be placed well back from the wound edge to avoid this zone.[10]

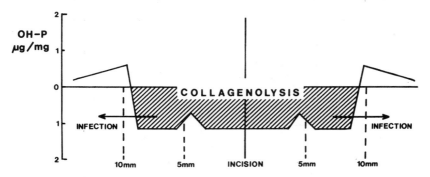

FIG. 2. *The chemically active zone of an incised wound extends for at least 5 mm on either side. Collagen lysis is prominent in the first week and is even more marked when infection is present. (After Adamsons RJ et al: Surg Gynecol Obstet 123:515, 1966)*

THE SUTURES

Sutures are foreign bodies and as such may adversely affect wound healing.[11,12,13] There are three principle considerations.

First, there is the amount of suture material implanted. This is most readily minimized by using the finest sutures at all times (Fig. 3). The metallic sutures are the strongest, and natural sutures, such as silk and catgut, are the weakest.[14] The synthetic materials, which lie in between, are usually selected because they are, in general, easier to use than the metals. Since the volume of implanted material rises with the square of the diameter (Fig. 4), one size heavier than necessary results in a significantly greater amount of material being left in a wound.[10] It makes little sense to use a suture of a strength much greater than that of the tissue it is holding. Indeed, most tissues are remarkably weak and only in the condensed collagen layers does holding power approach that of 1-0 chromic catgut. Elsewhere a finer suture will suffice.

The second point is the lack of relationship between absorbability and suture strength. Absorbable sutures lose strength rapidly and provide little effective support after a month (Fig. 5).[15] Despite this, the suture may persist, apparently intact, for 90 days or more; it continues

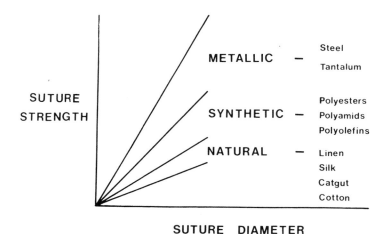

SUTURE   DIAMETER

FIG. 3. *The strength of a suture determines the size that is used. Natural fibers are the weakest and metallic ones are the strongest. The synthetics lie between and provide a fine suture of high strength. When they are used, less foreign material is implanted in the wound.*

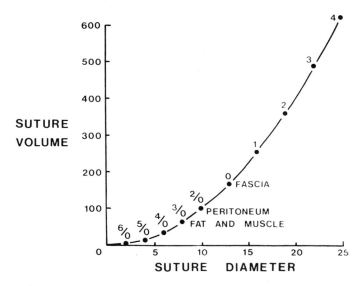

FIG. 4. *The volume of implanted material goes up with the square of the diameter and selection of a suture one size heavier than necessary results in significantly more material being left behind in the wound.*

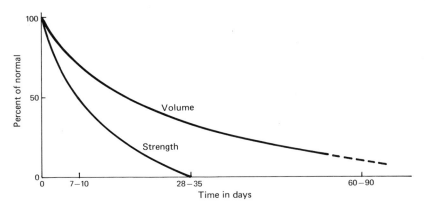

FIG. 5. *Absorbable sutures loose strength much more quickly than they are absorbed. After one month they provide little if any support, although they continue to act as a foreign body.*

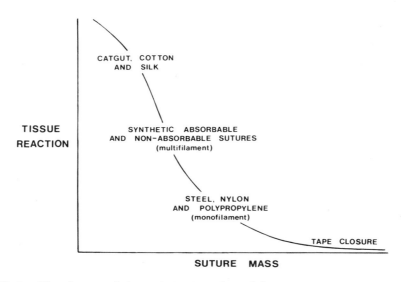

FIG. 6.   *The degree of tissue irritation elicited by a suture is an important determinant of wound infection. In general the natural materials are the most irritating and the synthetic monofilaments the least.*

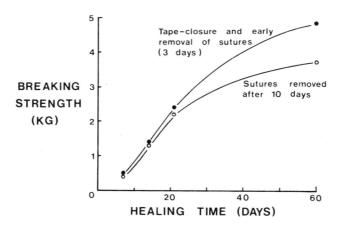

FIG. 7.   *Wounds sutured with silk do not recover as much strength as adjacent tape-closed wounds. The impaired strength is a consequsnce of tissue irritation and is avoided by removing sutures at 3 days instead of at 10. (After Brunius U: Acta Chir Scand [Supp] 395, 1968)*

to be a foreign body without helping support the wound. On this basis it is hard to advocate its use when infection seems likely.

The third point is the extent to which the particular suture irritates the tissues. All sutures elicit some degree of inflammatory response (Fig. 6).[16,17,18] In general, natural materials are the most troublesome and synthetic monofilaments the least. The braided synthetics, whether absorbable or nonabsorbable, have an intermediate position. The irritative effect delays healing (Fig. 7).[12] and enhances the infectivity of pathogens.[13] Although this effect is minimized by using bland monofilaments,[11] it is not entirely eliminated until sutures are dispensed with and the wound closed with tape.[19,20,21]

PRACTICAL ASPECTS OF WOUND REPAIR

Given the fact that the wound is a delicate tissue which recovers strength slowly and is surrounded by a softened zone of normal tissue, how do we select the appropriate sutures for a given situation?

The Contaminated Wound

Nearly all surgical wounds are contaminated with pathogenic bacteria but few become septic; wounds have an innate ability to resist infection.[22] Infection cannot occur without bacteria, but it seems that in about half the cases local enhancing factors determine the outcome. Of these, devitalized tissue and foreign material are the principal offenders. Although a single piece of silk suture enhances the infectivity of pathogens to a remarkable degree, the real damage is done by the focal necrosis produced by tying it (Fig. 8)[13] It makes good sense, therefore, to avoid sutures in a contaminated wound and let it heal by second intention.[23,24,25] As an alternative, primary closure can be delayed for four or five days until granulation tissue has developed. There is then very little risk of an invasive infection developing, and the overall healing time is only marginally prolonged.[21,26] If sutures are required, bland, synthetic monofilament materials are to be preferred for the deeper tissues, but tape closure should still be chosen where possible.[19,20,21,23]

The other useful measures are directed at the bacteria. Prompt administration of appropriate antibiotics or antiseptics can cut the infection rate in half.[27-32] Therapy must be started as soon as possible and is ineffective if delayed more than an hour or two. For the same reason, treatment is not prolonged and questions of toxicity and resistant strains are largely irrelevant. Our routine is to give a 1 gm intra-

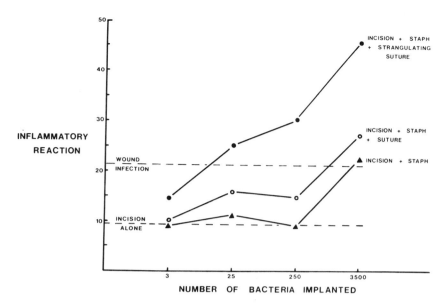

FIG. 8. *The presence of extraneous material in a wound enhances the likelihood of infection developing. The effect of tying a suture is particularly dramatic. (After Howe C: Surg Gynecol Obstet 123:507, 1966)*

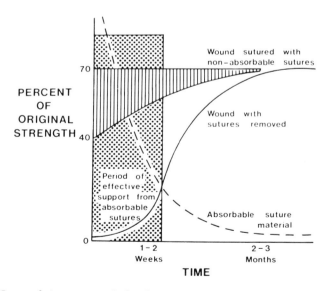

FIG. 9. *Strength is recovered slowly in fascial wounds and suture support is required for about 3 months. The moment a wound is sutured it has between 40 and 70 percent of its original strength. This is maintained when nonabsorbable sutures are used. Absorbable sutures lose their strength before the wound has fully recovered and dehiscence is more likely.*

venous bolus of a cephalosporin as soon as possible after contamination. A second dose five hours later appears to be useful, but a third is almost certainly unnecessary.

Fascial Wounds

The moment a fascial wound is sutured it has between 40 and 70 percent of the strength of unwounded tissue (Fig. 9).[33,34,35] The wound itself has little strength during the first few weeks and during this period absorbable sutures lose almost all their supporting capacity. If they are used as the sole means of repair, the wound is critically weak when most patients are being actively mobilized. At present the only way to prolong suture support is by selecting nonabsorbable materials.

Fascial Repair

The midline incision provides quick and easy access to the abdomen and dehiscence can virtually be eliminated when the particular characteristics of the wound and suture are borne in mind. The requirements are gentle prolonged support with a minimum amount of non-irritating material. A continuous synthetic monofilament fits these requirements, and wide spacing of the bites insures they are safely outside the lytic zone. Although the suture is weak where knotted, serious loss of strength only occurs where it is inadvertently nipped with a metal instrument. This technical point is easily learned and the closure has proved effective in a series of over 250 consecutive midline closures. Two wound failures have occurred and these were due to the sutures "cutting out" following prolonged local wound infection. In both cases the simple over-and-over technique appeared to have been responsible and we have adopted the more secure mattress repair. In other respects infection is not a problem; as long as the knots are buried, granulation tissue grows over an exposed synthetic monofilament suture and healing progresses to completion without the necessity of disturbing the suture.[36] This insures that support is maintained throughout healing. An important technical point is to close the peritoneum separately and avoid the rare but serious problems associated with intra-abdominal suture loops.

The Resutured Wound

When a dehisced wound is resutured it usually heals remarkably well.[37,38] Experiments show that this is because it has a head start (Fig.

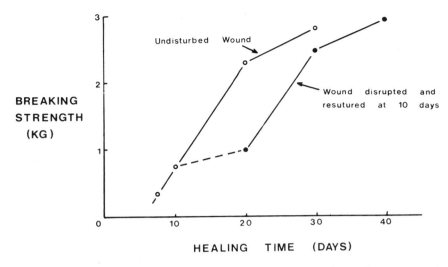

FIG. 10. *If a healing wound is broken open and resutured it picks up strength rapidly. Ten days later it is stronger than a fresh 10-day wound, but still a good deal weaker than if it had been left undisturbed.*

10). Local healing changes are well established and the resutured wound is not comparable to a fresh one.[39] These active local changes persist for a month or two and it therefore makes good sense to operate through the first wound if a second operation is required during that period.

Repair of Special Tissues

The relative importance of the components of healing varies from one site to another. Anastomoses in bowel, urinary tract, and blood vessels present special requirements:

Bowel
   rapid collagen turnover
   prolonged suture support (helpful)
Urinary tract
   rapid healing
   absorbable sutures
Blood vessels
   limited scar tissue
   prolonged suture support (mandatory)

In the gastrointestinal tract a flexible, leakproof repair is sought.[40] No great strength is required, and since healing is rapid the well-known problems with colonic anastomosis are, at first sight, a little surprising. This puzzle has now been clarified. Collagen has an unusually high turnover rate in healing colon. Collagenase activity is high, and during the first four to six days up to 40 percent of the old collagen is removed from either side of the wound.[41,42,43] Fortunately, strength is usually well maintained by the rapid synthesis of new collagen. The balance, however, is easily upset by local factors such as trauma, foreign material, and bacterial contamination.[44,45] Leakage is minimized by protecting the wound from destructive forces, such as distension, and by providing continued support with fine nonirritant, nonabsorbable sutures.

In the urinary tract healing is again rapid. Although anastomotic leaking may occur it is rarely a threat to life. The use of nonabsorbable sutures is not justifiable since they are associated with a high incidence of concretion formation.

In blood vessels the connective tissue response is limited[46] and anastomotic leaking is unacceptable. Suture support is required indefinitely. Special care is needed in the heart and major blood vessels; since intraluminal pressures are high and the wound is additionally stressed by the further assaults of about 40 million heartbeats per year, synthetic, totally nonabsorbable sutures are mandatory.

Skin Closure

When fascial closure is secure, skin repair need not be particularly strong and management is directed towards preventing wound infection and leaving a cosmetically acceptable scar. Wound infection is primarily a subcutaneous problem since these tissues offer little resistance to infection and pus accumulation. When contamination is severe, it is best to treat the wound by delayed primary closure or by allowing it to heal by second intention. When contamination is less severe, it is sufficient to avoid percutaneous suture and use surgical tape to approximate the wound edges.[19,20] In cases of technical difficulty, a continuous subcuticular stitch is the answer. Ideally, this should be removed by the second or third day to avoid any local irritating effects.[12,47] In practice, monofilaments like polypropylene are so bland that this is of little moment. The end result is cosmetically good, but the marked diminution of wound pain and edema is particularly beneficial. Patients move around readily and the usual problems associated with immobility are notable by their absence.

SUMMARY

A wound heals itself by means of connective tissue derived from a delicate system of cells and capillaries. Strength is recovered very slowly and prolonged suture support may therefore be necessary. This should be a gentle corseting to insure wound perfusion and oxygenation. Security is improved by inserting the stitches well outside the wound edge, which can soften unpredictably.

In skin, percutaneous sutures are best avoided since surgical tape closure with or without subcuticular support is associated with better overall results. Elsewhere a fine synthetic material should be selected.

The single most important factor in determining the outcome, however, is good surgical technique.[5,48] When this is absent the other recommendations count for little.

REFERENCES

1. Hunt TK, Zederfeldt B, Goldstick TK: Oxygen and healing. Am J Surg 118:521, 1969
2. Silver IA: The measurement of oxygen tension in healing tissue. Prog Resp Res 3:124, 1969
3. Hunt TK, Pai MP: The effect of varying ambient oxygen tensions on wound metabolism and collagen synthesis. Surg Gynecol Obstet 135:561, 1972
4. Hunt TK, Linsey M, Sonne M, Jawetz E: Oxygen tension and wound infection. Surg Forum 23:47, 1972
5. Dykes ER, Anderson R: Atraumatic technic—The sine qua non of operative wound infection prophylaxis. Clev Clin 28:157, 1961
6. Niinikoski J: Effect of oxygen supply on wound healing and formation of experimental granulation tissue. Acta Physiol Scand [Suppl] 334, 1969
7. Niinikoski J, Hunt TK, Dunphy JE: Oxygen supply in healing tissue. Am J Surg 123:247, 1972
8. Douglas DM: The healing of aponeurotic incisions. Br J Surg 40:79, 1952
9. Adamsons RJ, Musco F, Enquist IF: The chemical dimensions of a healing incision. Surg Gynecol Obstet 123:515, 1966
10. Forrester JC: Suture materials and their use. Brit J Hosp Med 8:578, 1972
11. Alexander JW, Kaplan JZ, Altemeier WA: Role of suture materials in the development of wound infections. Ann Surg 165:192, 1967
12. Brunius U: Wound healing impairment from sutures. Acta Chir Scand [Suppl] 395, 1968
13. Howe CW: Experimental studies on determinants of wound infection. Surg Gynecol Obstet 123:507, 1966
14. Herrmann JB: Tensile strength and knot security of surgical suture materials. Am Surg 37:209, 1971
15. Lawrie P, Angus GE, Reese AJM: The absorption of surgical catgut. Br J Surg 47:551, 1960
16. Madsen ET: An experimental and clinical evaluation of surgical suture materials—I & II. Surg Gynecol Obstet 97:73 & 439, 1953

17. Madsen ET: An experimental and clinical evaluation of surgical suture materials—III. Surg Gynecol Obstet 106:216, 1958
18. Postlethwait RW: Tissue reaction to surgical sutures. In Dunphy JE, Van Winkle HW (eds): Repair and Regeneration. New York, McGraw-Hill,1969
19. Conolly WB, Hunt TK, Dunphy JE: Management of contaminated surgical wounds. Surg Gynecol Obstet 129:593, 1969
20. Dunphy JE, Jackson DS: Practical applications of experimental studies in the care of the primarily closed wound. Am J Surg 104:273, 1962
21. Edlich RF, Rogers W, Kasper G, et al: Studies in the management of the contaminated wound, I & II. Am J Surg 117: 323, 1969
22. Altemeier WA, Todd JC: Studies on the incidence of infection following open chest cardiac massage for cardiac arrest. Ann Surg 158:596, 1963
23. Carpendale MTF, Sereda W: The role of the percutaneous suture in surgical wound infection. Surgery 58:672, 1965
24. Grosfeld JL, Solit RW: Prevention of wound infection in perforated appendicitis: Experience with delayed primary wound closure. Ann Surg 168:891, 1968
25. Wilkie DPD: Appendicitis. Ann Surg 100:202, 1934
26. Shepard GH: The healing of wounds after delayed primary closure. An experimental study. Plast Reconst Surg 48:358, 1971
27. Belzer FO, Salvatierra O, Schweizer RT, Kountz SM: Prevention of wound infections by topical antibiotics in high risk patients. Am J Surg 126:180, 1973
28. Burke JF: Wound infection and early inflammation. Monogr Surg Sci 1:301, 1964
29. Evans C, Pollock AV: The reduction of surgical wound infections by prophylactic parenteral cephaloridine. Br J Surg 60:434, 1973
30. Gilmore OJA, Martin TDM, Fletcher BN: Prevention of wound infection after appendicetomy. Lancet 1:220, 1973
31. Mountain JC, Seal PV: Topical ampicillin in grid-iron appendicectomy wounds. Br J Clin Pract 24:111, 1970
32. Polk HC, Lopez-Mayor JF: Postoperative wound infection: A prospective study of determinant factors and prevention. Surg 66:97, 1969
33. Adamsons RJ, Enquist IF: The relative importance of sutures to the strength of healing wounds under normal and abnormal conditions. Surg Gynecol Obstet 117:396, 1963
34. Howes EL: The immediate strength of the sutured wound. Surgery 7:24, 1940
35. Lichtenstein IL, Herzikoff S, Shore JM, et al: The dynamics of wound healing. Surg Gynecol Obstet 130:685, 1970
36. Everett WG: Suture materials in general surgery. Prog Surg 8:14, 1970
37. Douglas DM: Acceleration of wound healing produced by preliminary wounding. Br J Surg 46:401, 1959
38. Savlov ED, Dunphy JE: The healing of the disrupted and resutured wound. Surgery 36:362, 1954
39. Madden JW, Smith HC: The rate of collagen synthesis and deposition in dehisced and resutured wounds. Surg Gynecol Obstet 130:487, 1970
40. Van Winkle W, Hastings JC: Considerations in the choice of suture material for various tissues. Surg Gynecol Obstet 135:113, 1972
41. Cronin K, Jackson DS, Dunphy JE: Changes in bursting strength and collagen content of the healing colon. Surg Gynecol Obstet 126:747, 1968

42. Cronin K, Jackson DS, Dunphy JE: Specific activity of hydroxyproline—Tritium in the healing colon. Surg Gynecol Obstet 126:1061, 1968

43. Hawley PR, Faulk WP, Hunt TK, Dunphy JE: Collagenase activity in the gastro-intestinal tract. Br J Surg 57:896, 1970

44. Hunt TK, Hawley PR: Surgical judgment and colonic anastomoses. Dis Colon Rectum 12:167, 1969

45. Irvin TT, Goligher JC: Aetiology of disruption of colonic anastomoses. Br J Surg 60:461, 1973

46. Berger K, Sauvage LR, Rao AM, Wood SJ: Healing of arterial prostheses in man: Its incompleteness. Ann Surg 175:118, 1972

47. Myers MB, Cherry G, Heimberger S: Augmentation of wound tensile strength by early removal of sutures. Am J Surg 117:338, 1969

48. Condie JD, Ferguson DJ: Experimental wound infections: Contamination versus surgical technique. Surgery 50:367, 1961

Comment

Surgeons have argued for a century and a half about the proper choice of suture materials. As Mr. Forrester implies, the way the suture is used if often more important than the choice of the material. Due to many ancillary advances, "wound risk" is, in general, less than it used to be. It is no longer necessary to use thick sutures. In fact, as he points out, finer sutures gently tied are much preferable.

Mr. Forrester gives a good common sense guide to suture use. The argument over interrupted versus continuous suture lines still is on, and no one has proved superiority of one over the other. The running or continuous suture has the fault that if one part of it breaks, it all breaks but it has the advantage of speed and of having a self-adjusting tension. The interrupted suture requires more skill to tie each suture at just the right tension and leaves more suture in the wound, but the loss of one suture is rarely critical. With the exception of this one point, it would be difficult to argue with any part of this chapter.

Skin Closure: Sutures and Tape
16

Juhani Ahonen, Hasse Jiborn, and Bengt Zederfeldt

Coaption of wound surfaces is necessary to provide conditions for primary wound healing. In most situations sutures are required to obtain such approximation. However, since sutures are foreign bodies with potentially negative effects on the healing process (Brunius 1968; van Winkle and Hastings 1972; Postlethwait et al. 1975) there are reasons to avoid sutures for wound closure whenever possible, adhesive tape offering a preferable alternative.

Wound closure without sutures has been practiced for thousands of years but advantages and problems with this technique have been thoroughly penetrated only during the last decades. Wounds closed by tape and by suture differ as regards inflammatory reaction, infection rate, mechanical properties, and cosmetic results. The aim of this chapter is to discuss the relative merits of tape and sutures for skin-wound closure.

INFLAMMATORY REACTION

The inflammatory reaction in a wound is caused by the injury to the tissues and by foreign bodies present in the wound area. Increased trauma by the passing of needles and sutures and the presence of suture material exaggerates and/or prolongs the inflammatory reaction in the wound region. In histologic studies Gillman et al. (1955) demonstrated that the inflammatory reaction is less pronounced in wounds closed by tape than in wounds closed by suture. Brunius et al. (1967) confirmed these findings and demonstrated a prolongation of the inflammatory reaction when sutures were used. Wounds from which sutures were removed 3 days after closure showed no increase in inflammation compared with tape-closed wounds (Brunius and Åhrén 1968a, b). This indicates that the early inflammatory reaction is a consequence of the injury and that the presence of sutures in the wound area after the third day prolongs the inflammatory reaction.

INFECTION RATE

Host defense against invading bacteria is markedly impaired by foreign body present in the tissues (e.g., Elek 1956), and it has shown experimentally that sutures increase the risk of infection in wounds with critical bacterial contamination (Edlich et al. 1973). In clinical studies it has been shown that skin closure by tape significantly diminishes the rate of wound infection in clean-contaminated and contaminated wounds while the infection rate in clean wounds is independent of the method of closure (e.g., Conolly et al. 1969).

Thus, experimental and clinical studies indicate that skin closure by tape reduces the risk of infection in wounds with critical bacterial contamination.

MECHANICAL PROPERTIES

Brunius et al. (1967, 1968) found higher breaking strength in tape-closed than in sutured rat skin incisions from 7 to 60 days after wounding (Fig. 1). Forrester et al. (1970) likewise found tape-closed wounds to be stronger than sutured wounds late in the healing process (20 to 150 days), but could not verify increased strength of tape-closed wounds in the early healing period (Fig. 2). The different results in the earlier periods might result from different techniques for strength determinations. While Brunius et al. determined breaking strength *in situ* Forrester and co-workers studied excised wounds.

Brunius et al. ascribed their findings of higher breaking strength during the early phase of healing to lesser inflammatory reaction in the tape-closed wounds.

The higher strength of tape-closed wounds in the later stages of healing seems to be a consequence of increased tension over the wound due to retraction of the divided subcutaneous muscle. Myers et al. 1969 have demonstrated that increased tension within certain limits increases strength development in wounds. Forrester et al. (1970) demonstrated the different architectures of the collagen structure in tape-closed and sutured wounds. The alignment of the fibrils was more pronounced in the tape-closed wounds than in the sutured wounds. This difference, which may be an effect of tension, readily explains higher strength of tape-closed wounds. Support for this explanation was further found in studies in which the subcutaneous muscle was left intact (Brunius et al. 1968). When tension was thus avoided there were no differences in late strength of tape-closed wounds as compared to sutured wounds.

In a thorough analysis of the mechanical properties of tape-closed and suture-closed skin incisions Forrester et al. (1970) found that energy absorption was the same in tape-closed and sutured wounds. The tape-closed wounds showed less extensibility than the sutured wounds. The interpretation of these findings is that tape closure results in scars that have higher strength but are slightly more brittle.

These differences in the mechanical properties of tape-closed and

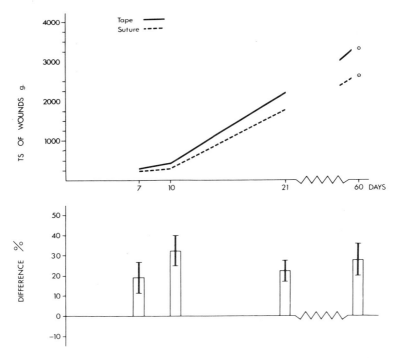

FIG. 1. Strength development in tape closed and sutured wounds from 7 to 60 days. The upper part shows the strength of the wounds. The lower part shows the percentage difference in strength between tape-closed and sutured wounds. (From Brunius et al. 1967)

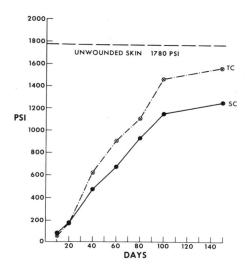

FIG. 2. Tensile strength of rat skin wounds closed by tape (TC) and suture (SC) from 10 to 150 days after wounding. (From Forrester et al. 1970)

sutured wounds, although they are of considerable theoretical interest, probably have minor or no importance in practice. It is not possible to conclude that tape closure has advantages over suture closure with respect to mechanical properties of the scar as we do not know that a scar with higher breaking strength and lower extensibility is preferable to a scar with lower breaking strength and higher extensibility.

COSMETIC RESULTS

Avoidance of suture marks is one obvious advantage of tape closure. With tape closure, however, it is often difficult to obtain and maintain perfect adaptation of the wound edges even if especially difficult areas with hair, concave surfaces, etc., are avoided. In our experience there is no general cosmetic advantage of tape closure of wounds over suture closure especially if sutures are removed early and stitch marks are thus avoided.

PRACTICAL CONSIDERATIONS

The principle of using skin closure by tape to avoid foreign bodies in the tissues is biologically sound; the main advantage of tape closure is decreased infection rate in wounds with critical bacterial contamination. One problem with tape closure is the difficulty in obtaining perfect adaptation of wound edges, which often results in less than perfect cosmetic results.

Since sutures seem to exert their negative effects when present in tissues for more than three days (Brunius 1968), a practical way of wound closure is as follows: fine monofilament synthetic sutures are used for wound closure; sutures are removed at three days and the wound from then on supported by tape. The advantages are that (1) perfect adaptation is insured, (2) the cosmetic result is good with stitch marks avoided, (3) the infection rate is still less, and (4) patients need not be seen as outpatients for the sole purpose of suture removal.

REFERENCES

Brunius U: Wound healing impairment from sutures. Acta Chir Scand [Suppl] 395, 1968

Brunius U, Åhrén C: Healing during the cicatrization phase of skin incisions closed by non-suture technique. Acta Chir Scand 135:289, 1968a

Brunius U, Åhrén C: Healing impairment in skin incisions closed with silk sutures. Acta Chir Scand 135:369, 1968b

Brunius U, Zederfeldt B, Åhrén C: Healing of skin incisions closed by non-suture technique. Acta Chir Scand 133:509, 1967

Brunius U, Zederfeldt B, Åhrén C: Healing of skin incisions with intact subcutaneous muscle closed by non-suture technique. Acta Chir Scand 134:187, 1968

Conolly WB, Hunt TK, Zederfeldt B, Cafferata HT, Dunphy JE: Clinical comparison of surgical wounds closed by suture and adhesive tapes. Am J Surg 117:318, 1969

Edlich RF, Panek PH, Rodeheaver GT, Turnbull VG, Kurtz LD, Edgerton MT: Physical and chemical configuration of sutures in the development of surgical infection. Ann Surg 177:679, 1973

Elek SD: Experimental staphylococcal infections in the skin of man. Ann NY Acad Sci 65:85, 1956

Forrester JC, Zederfeldt BH, Hayes TL, Hunt TK: Tape-closed and sutured wounds: a comparison by tensiometry and scanning electron microscopy. Br J Surg 57:729, 1970

Gillman T, Penn J, Bronks D, Roux M: Closure of wounds and incisions with adhesive tape. Lancet 269:2, 945, 1955

Myers MB, Cherry G, Heimburger S: Augmentation of wound tensile strength by early removal of sutures. Am J Surg 117:338, 1969

Postlethwait RW, Willigan DA, Ulin AW: Human tissue reaction to sutures. Ann Surg 181:144, 1975

van Winkle W, Hastings H: Considerations in the choice of suture material for various tissues. Collective review. Surg Gynecol Obstet 135:113, 1972

Comment

Herein is summarized the relevant literature on the closure of skin with tapes. The authors have purposefully not cited the entire literature but such lists are available.

One of the mysteries of our time, it seems to me, is why this simple, effective, sensible, inexpensive techique has taken so long to achieve widespread use. One might understand if tapes regularly fell off or broke; but they don't. All reports agree that when used appropriately, tapes are as good as sutures, except that they are more economical, hurt less, require less attention, and lessen the incidence of infection.

Like any other technique, there are limitations. Tapes don't hold on bloody, wet wounds. The presence of hair discourages their use. Loose, wrinkled skin is a relative contraindication. The decisions, however, are not difficult, and simple common sense is enough to guide the surgeon's judgment.

The Biology of Infections: Sutures, Tapes, and Bacteria

17

Richard F. Edlich, George Rodeheaver, Gerald T. Golden, and Milton T. Edgerton

Since every surgical wound is contaminated to some degree by micro-organisms, a surgical operation is, in fact, an exercise in surgical microbiology. The ultimate outcome of a surgical wound hangs in a delicate balance between the causal factors of infection (the number and virulence of the pathogen) and the host's resistance to infection. The most important determinant of infection often is the number of bacteria in the wound. A critical number of bacteria is necessary to elicit suppuration that will disrupt the wound edges. This number is usually very large (10^6 or more organisms per gram of tissue) since the host's tissues normally offer considerable resistance to infection. When the host's defenses are impaired for any reason, fewer bacteria can cause clinically significant suppuration.

Undoubtedly, the most common reason for impaired resistance is inadequate surgical techniques. Studies have shown that a single suture in the wound interferes with tissue resistance against infection, and this is due to several factors.[1,2] The quantity of suture material is very important. Thick sutures invite more infection than thin ones and long sutures more than short.

The chemical structure of a suture has a significant influence on the development of infection. Utilizing a standardized experimental model,[2] we noted that the infection-potentiating effects of nylon and polypropylene sutures were less than that of any other nonabsorbable suture. Multifilament natural fiber (silk and cotton) sutures potentiated infection more than any other suture. The potentiation by Dacron and stainless steel was intermediate between those of the synthetic and natural-fiber sutures.

Among the absorbable sutures, polyglycolic acid (PGA) sutures evoked the least inflammatory response and were comparable to nylon and polypropylene sutures. The infection-potentiating effects of PGA were significantly less than gut. *In vitro* studies performed in our laboratory indicated that the degradation products of the polyglycolic acid sutures and nylon sutures are potent antibacterials.[2] It is postulated that the degradation products of these sutures may destroy some of the bacteria in the wound.

Surprisingly, the physical configuration of the suture plays a relatively unimportant role in the development of early experimental infection. Although the infection-potentiating effect of monofilament, nonabsorbable sutures in contaminated tissues was less than that of multifilament sutures made of the same material, these differences were neither large nor statistically significant.

Gentleness in handling tissues has been found to be mandatory in closing the contaminated wound. Sutures tied tightly around wound edges markedly increase the incidence of wound infection because of the strangulation of tissue within the suture loop and its associated lowering of the host's defenses. However, the infection-potentiating effect of the least reactive suture is apparent even when the best atraumatic technique is employed. This damaging effect of sutures is particularly apparent in certain clinical settings.

PERCUTANEOUS SUTURES

Percutaneous sutures, in a sense, penetrate the host's defenses against infection.[3] Their deleterious effects can be evaluated by employing graded bacterial inocula in experimental wounds subjected to either suture or tape closure techniques. By recording the inflammatory responses of these wounds to various inocula, dose response curves were constructed (Fig. 1). When the level of contamination was 10^4 organisms or less, the incidence of infection in the wounds approximated by the least reactive nonabsorbable suture (5-0 monofilament nylon) was comparable with that of wounds closed by tape *without* sutures. This degree of contamination is often found in clean, elective surgical procedures.

For wounds contaminated with 10^5 or 10^6 bacteria, the wound infecton rate was related to the closure technique. The infection rate of the sutured wounds was significantly higher than that of taped wounds ($p < 0.05$). This level of contamination is comparable to that which occurs as a result of elective surgery in which the gastrointestinal tract has been opened. When 10^7 bacteria were applied to wounds, infection

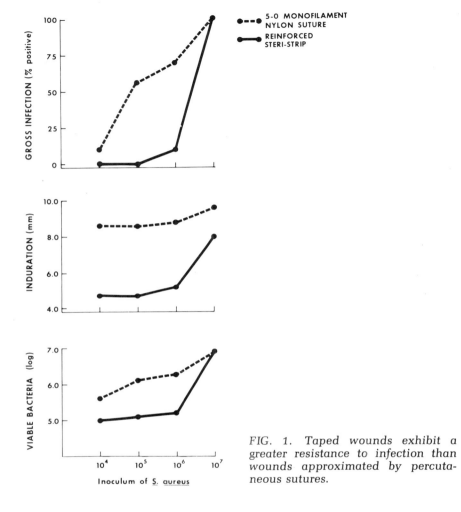

FIG. 1. *Taped wounds exhibit a greater resistance to infection than wounds approximated by percutaneous sutures.*

developed regardless of the closure technique. This level of inoculum is similar to that present in wounds contracted by pus or known infected fluid during an operation. Primary closure of such wounds invariably results in infection, and therefore delayed primary closure of the skin and subcutaneous tissue is mandatory.

The number of viable bacteria recovered from taped wounds was lower than that found in sutured wounds in all groups except those receiving 10^7 *Staphylococcus aureus*. In this latter group, the number of viable bacteria recovered from both wounds was not significantly

different. Taped wounds were able to resist bacterial growth more effectively than sutured wounds.

SUBCUTANEOUS SUTURES

Many surgeons believe that failure to close the subcutaneous adipose
tissue results in a dead space which predisposes the wound to infection, and closure of subcutaneous adipose tissue by an absorbable suture is commonly practiced. The influence of this technique on the
development of infection was investigated in an experimental model
using the domestic swine, which has a thick layer of adipose tissue
comparable to that found in humans. Even when the least reactive
absorbable suture (polyglycolic acid, 5-0) was used, closure of the
subcutaneous layer potentiated the development of infection (Fig. 2).
In wounds contaminated with 10^5 bacteria, the infection rate of the
wounds subjected to suture closure of dead space was 62 percent,
while there were no infections in the wounds in which subcutaneous
tissue was not approximated by suture. In those receiving 10^6 bacteria,
all wounds subjected to subcutaneous closure were infected, while
only 25 percent of the wounds without closure of the subcutaneum
were infected. The mean bacterial counts of these wounds with closure
were significantly higher than those wounds without closure of subcutaneous tissue at both levels of inoculum. It would appear that suture
closure of adipose tissue should be avoided in the contaminated, taped

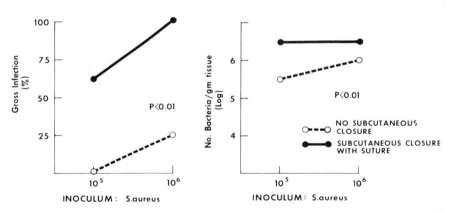

FIG. 2.   *Suture closure (5-0 polyglycolic acid) of adipose tissue in taped
wounds impairs the tissue's ability to resist infection and enhances bacterial
growth.*

wound. An incision through the subcutaneum does not inevitably cause a sizable "dead space." In fact, simple incision rarely does—even in the obese.

TAPE CLOSURE

The superior resistance to infection offered by taped as compared with sutured wounds in our studies suggests that tape closure of contaminated wounds is a significant clinical tool. A variety of tapes are available to the surgeon for a sutureless wound closure, including a cloth tape, Ethistrips (Ethicon, Inc.), a nonwoven microporous tape, Steristrips (3M Company), and a nonwoven microporous reinforced tape, Reinforced Steri-strips (3M Company). Each is composed of a tape backing and a chemical adhesive. The backing supports the adhesive and distributes tension over the entire tape surface; it is composed of tightly woven rayon fibers (Fig. 3). The tightness of the weave limits the number and size of the pores between the fiber interstices. The adhesive is a uniform polyalkylacrylate with relatively few interruptions in its continuity (2000 pores/sq in). The backing of the nonwoven microporous tape has multiple fine rayon fibers distributed randomly (Fig. 4). Numerous micropores are apparent between the fibers, forming continuous channels that pass from the surface of the backing to the adhesive. The adhesive is a discontinuous layer of polyalkylacrylate containing approximately 5000 pores/sq in.

The development of the newer nonwoven, reinforced, microporous tape necessitated two changes in the configuration of the nonwoven tape (Fig. 5). Longitudinal rayon fiber bundles were passed beneath the nonwoven fiber backing to enhance its strength. In addition, a "tackifier" was added to the hypoallergenic adhesive to improve adhesion. These structural modifications did not alter the tape's microporous structure (5000 pores/sq in). Maintenance of its microporous structure insures the passage of gas and water vapor through the tape.

The composition of a tape as well as its physical configuration influences its performance considerably. The performance of a tape can be characterized by its adhesive, tensile strength, and porosity. A surgical tape's adhesive must be aggressive and provide a firm tape-to-skin bond. The rare skin separation occurs during or immediately after tape wound closure, when the adhesive bond of the tape to the skin is weakest. Twenty-four hours after taping, the adhesive bond to the skin is twofold stronger than immediately following application. The adhesive bond to skin of the cloth tape and nonwoven microporous tape

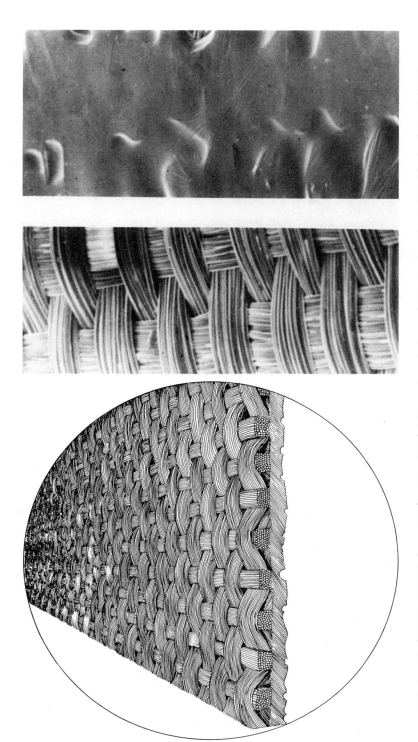

FIG. 3. Cloth tape. (Left) Schematic drawing. (Right) Scanning electron photomicrographs (×50). The backing of this tape (left) consists of tightly woven rayon fibers. The adhesive (right) beneath the backing is uniform with relatively few pores (2000 pores/sq in).

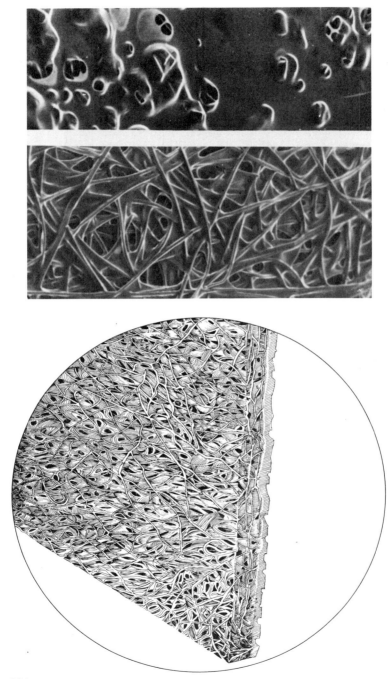

FIG. 4. Nonwoven microporous tape. (Left) Schematic drawing. (Right) Scanning electron microscope photographs (×40). The backing of this tape (left) contains multiple randomly distributed rayon fibers. Numerous micropores are apparent between the rayon fibers. The adhesive (right) is a discontinuous layer with numerous micropores throughout its surfaces (5000 pores/sq in).

220

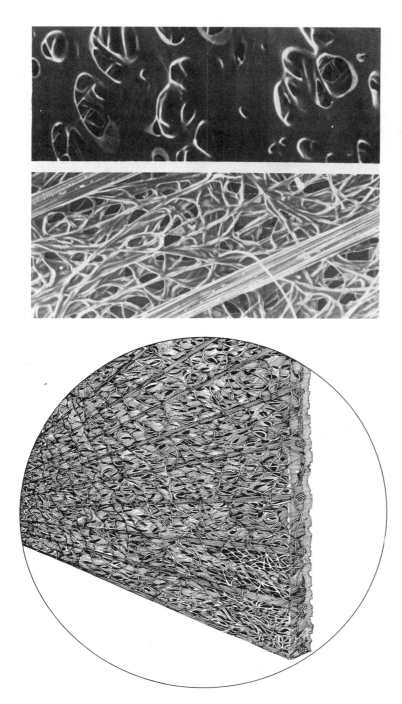

FIG. 5. Nonwoven, reinforced microporous tape. (Left) Schematic drawing. (Right) Scanning electron microscope photomicrographs (×40). Longitudinal rayon fiber bundles are passed beneath the nonwoven fiber backing (left) to increase the breaking strength of the tape. The addition of a tackifier to the adhesive (right) does not alter the porosity of the tape (5000 pores/sq in).

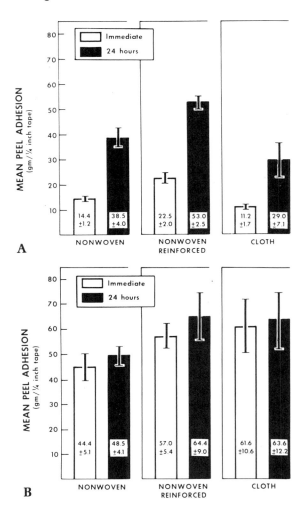

FIG. 6. *The mean peel adhesion of surgical tapes to (**A**) untreated human skin and (**B**) human skin subjected to an adhesive adjunct (tincture of benzoin).*

is weak, promoting immediate dislodgement from the wound (Fig. 6). The "tackifier" added to the adhesive of the nonwoven, microporous, reinforced tape markedly enhances the immediate adhesion of tape to dry skin.

Despite this advantage, even the reinforced tape will not adhere to wet skin. Drying with a gauze sponge often does not completely remove wet exudate and tape adhesion is impaired. This problem can be avoided by applying an adhesive adjunct (tincture of benzoin or others) to the skin prior to tape application. Such adjuncts enhance the immediate adhesion of all types of tapes to the skin (see Fig. 6). Inadvertent spillage of the adjunct impairs the wound's ability to resist infection.[4] To minimize the chance of spillage into the wound, the adhesive adjunct is applied in a thin film to the skin at the wound edge with an applicator stick.

A surgical tape must be strong enough to maintain wound approximation during healing (Fig. 7). Weak tapes may not be able to resist the pull of the wound edges and may tear. Weak paper tape has been strengthened by adding reinforcing rayon filaments to its backing, resulting in a fourfold increase in tensile strength. In a clinical trial in which these reinforced microporous tapes were utilized, tape breakage did not occur.

Irritation of the skin may occur with occlusive tapes. Tapes that limit moisture vapor transmission cause accumulation of fluid beneath the tape promoting tissue maceration and bacterial growth. Microporous tapes circumvent this difficulty by allowing moisture to escape through the interstices of the tape, resulting in a dry skin beneath the

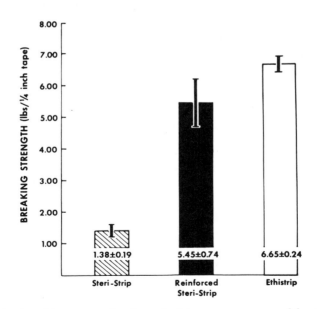

FIG. 7.   The breaking strength of surgical tapes as measured by the Instron Universal Testing Instrument.

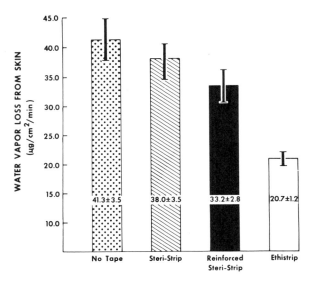

FIG. 8.   Measurement of transepidermal water loss through tapes as measured by electrohygrometry.

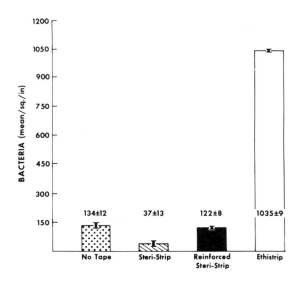

FIG. 9.   Bacterial growth under tapes applied to human skin.

tape which is antithetical to the growth of bacteria (Fig. 8). Cloth tape is occlusive because of its tightly woven cloth backing. This impairs the transmission of air and moisture vapor, encouraging bacterial growth (Fig. 9). This may have important clinical implications, particularly in the early phases of healing. Heavily contaminated moist skin under the cloth tape may be a potential source for infection in the incompletely epithelized wound.

RECOMMENDATIONS

The surgeon's choice of closure technique must be influenced by the degree of bacterial contamination in the wound. The majority of clean wounds will heal without infection regardless of the closure technique. In sharp contrast, the contaminated wound, in which a viscus has been opened, the choice of closure technique is critical. If percutaneous sutures are employed, infection is common. Tape closure of these wounds, however, can be done with minimal risk of infection. The benefit of tape closure in this group of patients has been reiterated by Conolly et al.[5] In their study, the incidence of gross infection in wounds closed by tape was significantly less (by about half!) than that in sutured wounds. Even the subcutaneous suture should be avoided in elective abdominal incisions, since they act as foreign bodies impairing the wound's ability to resist infection.

Contrary to the usual expectations, tape closure, without subcutaneous suture, is most easily accomplished in obese patients. The force necessary to approximate wound edges appears less than that in thin patients. In addition, the thick cut edge of adipose tissue tends to evert the skin, facilitating tape closure. In thin patients, supplemental interrupted subcuticular sutures may facilitate tape closure since they take the tension off the wound edge.

Primary closure of the skin and adipose tissue is *never* indicated in heavily contaminated wounds. In such wounds, contacted by pus or known infected fluid during the course of surgery, the number of bacteria deposited exceeds the infective dose and primary closure of such wounds will be followed inevitably by infection. In place of primary closure, delayed primary closure by tapes should be employed. The success of delayed primary closure in the treatment of the contaminated wound is an undisputed fact based on the reports of civilian and military surgeons.[6,7]

The technique of delayed closure of skin and subcutaneous tissue is important. Fine mesh gauze is placed (not packed!) between the cut edges of the tissue layers. The open wound is then covered by a sterile impervious dressing and is not inspected for the first four postoperative days unless the patient develops an unexplained fever. Inspection increases the risk of unavoidable contamination and subsequent infection. On or after the fifth postoperative day, the wound which appears uninfected can be approximated by tape with minimal risk of infection. This judgment can usually be made by inspection. Pus or excessive fibrin accumulation contraindicates closure.

The occasional wound that will develop infection following delayed closure may also be identified by utilizing quantitative microbiology. This technique consists of biopsying the wound 24 hours prior to closure and measuring the bacterial count by standard homogenization and dilution techniques. When the bacterial count of the tissue is 10^5 or less, delayed primary closure can be accomplished *without* risk of infection.[8] For wounds containing a higher level of inoculum, delayed primary closure is commonly followed by infection.

REFERENCES

1. Edlich RF, Tsung M-S, Rogers W, Rogers P, Wangensteen OH: Studies in management of the contaminated wound. I. Technique of closure of such wounds together with a note on a reproducible experimental model. J Surg Res 8:585, 1968
2. Edlich RF, Panek PH, Rodeheaver GT, Turnbull VG, Kurtz LD, Edgerton MT: Physical and chemical configuration of sutures in the development of surgical infection. Ann Surg 177:679, 1973
3. Edlich RF, Rodeheaver GT, Kuphal J, de Holl JD, Smith SL, Bacchetta C, Edgerton MT: Technique of closure: contaminated wounds. J Am Coll Emerg Phys 3:375, 1974
4. Panek PH, Prusak MP, Bolt D, Edlich RF: Potentiation of wound infection by adhesive adjuncts. Am Surg 38:343, 1972
5. Conolly WB, Hunt TK, Zederfeldt B, Cafferata HT, Dunphy JE: Clinical comparison of surgical wounds closed by suture and adhesive tapes. Am J Surg 117:318, 1969
6. Bernard HR, Cole WR: Wound infections following potentially contaminated operations. J Am Med Assoc 184:290, 1963
7. Heaton LD, Hughes CW, Rosegay H, Fisher GW, Feighny RE: Military surgical practices of the United States Army in Viet Nam. Curr Probl Surg, 1966, p 1
8. Robson MC, Hegger JP: Delayed wound closures based on bacterial counts. J Surg Oncol 2:379, 1970

Comment

Being the scientist he is, Dr. Edlich has probably understated his case. The importance of surgical technique in preventing infection probably cannot be overemphasized! Unfortunately, the well-known psychological effect, "condensation" of oft-repeated acts, tends to make bad surgeons of us all. Obviously, we usually "get away with" using sutures a size too large or using materials to which we are accustomed rather than newer and better materials. Since we usually get away with it, we repeat it until it becomes a habit, one which is often difficult to change. For instance, tape closure of skin has demonstrated its superiority over and over just as Dr. Edlich has reported. Yet, probably fewer than 10 percent of American surgeons use it! The cost in needless infections is immense! How often do you see heavy crushing clamps applied unnecessarily to fascia and subcutaneous tissue? How many surgeons use isolator drapes? How many overutilize electrocoagulation?

Recently, in the making of a training film, we wanted to include some examples of bad surgical technique. We couldn't film deliberately bad technique in humans for ethical reasons. We were thinking of using animals when our photographer, who has done many films for surgeons, suggested that he look through his "discarded" clippings file. With no difficulty at all, we found vivid examples of poor technique—all cut from films made by surgical leaders filming demonstrations of how certain operations should be done!

For reasons of sanity, surgeons ought to be allowed to forget a few infections in every hundred patients, and it is good that they can. If only we could keep infection figures for all surgeons so they could forget individual cases but be constantly reminded when their techniques are no longer adequate to their patients' needs. How many infections we could prevent! Most surgeons have about a 2 to 4 percent clean wound infection rate. These figures can be cut to 1 percent or 0.5 percent, but how many surgeons actually keep their figures and reach these goals?

In one small detail, I tend to disagree in practice (though not in principle) with Dr. Edlich. I tend to close primarily, with tapes, even contaminated wounds near stomas (though not those that have encountered pus or gross fecal spill). Delayed primary closures rarely succeed near a colostomy, and I can get more than 90 percent of such wounds to heal primarily without infection. Of course, one must be quick to open a questionably infected wound, but this is just a matter of diligence. On the whole, I feel I lower patient morbidity in this manner. The point of mentioning this is not to convert others to this practice, but to illustrate a principle: one often has the opportunity to decide what it is that one wants of the wound, and then get it!

Debridement: An Essential Component of Traumatic Wound Care

18

Beth Haury, George Rodeheaver, JoAnn Vensko, Milton T. Edgerton, and Richard F. Edlich

Debridement has been considered the most important single factor in the management of the contaminated wound.[1] This time-honored technique has two notable benefits. First, it removes tissue that is heavily contaminated by dirt and bacteria, protecting the patient from invasive infection.[2] Second, it removes devitalized tissues which impair the wound's ability to resist infection.[3,4] The purpose of this study is to quantitate the degree to which various devitalized soft tissues potentiated the development of infection in contaminated wounds. The results of this investigation provide the surgeon with insight into the consequences of inadequate debridement of contaminated soft-tissue wounds. In addition, the possible mechanisms by which devitalized tissue enhances infection were studied.

MATERIALS AND METHODS

Resistance to Infection

The purpose of this study was to ascertain the influence of devitalized soft tissue on the wound's ability to resist infection. Male guinea pigs of the Hartley strain (300–350 g) were selected as the experimental animal since they are susceptible to bacterial infection by the same organisms pathogenic to humans. Each animal was anesthetized with an intraperitoneal injection of sodium pentobarbital. The paravertebral hair was first removed by electric clippers followed by a razor. The skin was then washed with an iodophor solution followed by a 70 percent alcohol rinse. An aqueous solution of 1 percent sodium thiosulfate was then applied to the skin to inactivate residual iodine. The skin was then dried with a gauze sponge.

Following skin cleaning, devitalized tissue specimens were removed from animals immediately after sacrifice. Muscle samples were removed from paravertebral muscle by an aseptic technique. The fat pads located above the scapulae were the sources of fat specimens. The skin specimens were then harvested and either subjected to a standard thermal injury or remained untreated. A scald injury to designated skin samples was accomplished by immersing them in boiling water for 10 seconds.[5] A metal cylinder maintained at 375 C was applied to other skin samples for 5 seconds, rendering a full-thickness dry burn.[6]

After cleansing the skin of the animals in the remaining groups of animals, two standardized, paravertebral incisions measuring 3 cm in length were made in each animal. Each wound was then contaminated with a designated dose of *Staphylococcus aureus* (CDC* No. 2801) suspended in a measured volume (0.02 ml) of 0.9 percent saline. Ten minutes later one wound in each animal received a measured amount of a specific guinea pig soft tissue. Contralateral wounds served as a control for each animal and did not receive any tissue. All wounds were then closed with microporous tape.

The inflammatory responses of the wounds were recorded 4 days after wound closure. The width of the indurated margin of the wound was measured. The wounds were then opened and inspected for evidence of purulent discharge. A relative estimate of the bacteria in each wound was determined by standard serial dilution and culturing techniques.

Leukocyte Phagocytosis and Intracellular Kill

Traumatic injury and subsequent bacterial contamination elicit an inflammatory response. Alterations in the microvasculature occur that allow extravasation of phagocytic cells into the tissue. These cells possess the capacity to ingest and kill invading bacteria. Once a microorganism is phagocytized, it it normally destroyed by intracellular digestion. Microbial death does not always follow phagocytosis, however, and certain bacteria will survive within the leukocyte for prolonged

*Communicable Disease Center, Atlanta, Georgia.

periods of time. This phase of the study examined the effect of designated soft tissues on the ability of the leukocyte to phagocytize and kill bacteria.

In vitro measurement of leukocyte function was patterned after the technique described by Mandel and Vest.[7] Fresh venous blood collected in heparinized tubes was combined with an equal volume of 3 percent Dextran and placed at a 45° angle for 1 hour in order to sediment the erythrocytes. The supernatant containing plasma, leukocytes, and platelets was centrifuged at 280 g for 12 minutes and the resulting button of white blood cells (10^5) was resuspended in 3.4 ml of Hank's balanced salt solution and 0.4 ml of autologous serum. The fresh autologous serum contains the opsonins and complement system that facilitate phagocytosis of bacteria. One-half of the white cell suspensions received 10 mg/ml of a designated sample of homogenized tissue. The remaining cell suspensions served as controls and were not exposed to tissue. A measured aliquot (0.2 ml) of bacterial inoculum suspension (10^7) of S. aureus (ATCC* No. 12600) was added to both treated and control samples. The tubes were rotated at 12 rpm and maintained at 37 C.

Upon bacterial inoculation and at 2 hours postinoculation, a measured aliquot (0.1 ml) of fluid was removed from both test and control samples. This aliquot was diluted in sterile water (9.9 ml) and vortexed for 2 minutes in order to lyse the leukocytes. The total number of bacteria within the water was quantitated by standard serial dilution and plating techniques. The total number of bacteria represents those bacteria that were not phagocytized as well as those that were ingested but remained viable within the cell. Knowledge of the changes in the total number of bacteria within the 2-hour period of observation provides a measure of the bactericidal capacity of the leukocytes. Test results were calculated by the following equation and reported as log percent inhibition of bacterial kill:

$$\text{Log \% inhibition} = 100\% - 100 \frac{[\text{TEST}]}{[\text{CONTROL}]} \frac{\log \text{bacteria}_{0\,hr} - \log \text{bacteria}_{2hr}}{\log \text{bacteria}_{0\,hr} - \log \text{bacteria}_{2hr}}$$

In this phase of the study, the influence of devitalized fat on additional parameters of leukocyte function was ascertained. Suspensions

*American Type Culture Collection.

of white cells containing either 10 mg/ml of homogenized fat or devitalized tissue were inoculated with 10^7 S. aureus. Upon bacterial inoculation and at 1 and 2 hours postinoculation, a measured aliquot (0.5 ml) of fluid was removed from both test and control suspensions. This aliquot was diluted in sterile saline (4.5 ml). Through differential centrifugation (280 g), the free bacteria (supernatant) were separated from the leukocytes (sediment). After separating the sediment and supernatant, the leukocytes in the sediment were then lysed in sterile water in order to release any phagocytized yet viable bacteria. The number of free extracellular and intracellular bacteria was quantitated using standard serial dilution and plating techniques. Quantitation of extracellular bacteria (supernatant) over time provides an index of the actual bactericidal action within the leukocyte.

Bacterial Growth

In this portion of the study, the influence of devitalized soft tissue on bacterial growth was measured. Immediately after surgical excision of the soft-tissue specimens, a measured amount of each tissue (500 mg) was added to 4.5 ml of 0.9 percent sodium chloride. The tissue specimens were then homogenized for 3 minutes using a Polytron homogenizer. An aliquot (0.5 ml) of 0.9 percent sodium chloride containing 5.6×10^2 S. aureus was added to each homogenized suspension. A similar aliquot of bacterial inoculum was added to tubes containing 4.5 ml of trypticase soy broth without tissue serving as the controls. The tubes were gently rotated at 12 rpm in a 37 C incubator. Aliquots were removed at 1, 3, 5, 8, 12, and 18 hrs after incubation, and the number of viable bacteria determined by standard diluting and plating techniques.

RESULTS

Devitalized soft tissue damaged the host's resistance to infection. The infection rates of wounds containing devitalized tissue was significantly greater than the gross infection score for contralateral controls (Fig. 1). The degrees to which fat, muscle, and skin enhanced infection were comparable. The presence of purulent discharge in wounds containing devitalized tissue was associated with marked induration of the wound margin. Devitalized tissues encouraged the growth of bacteria as evidenced by the elevated bacterial counts.

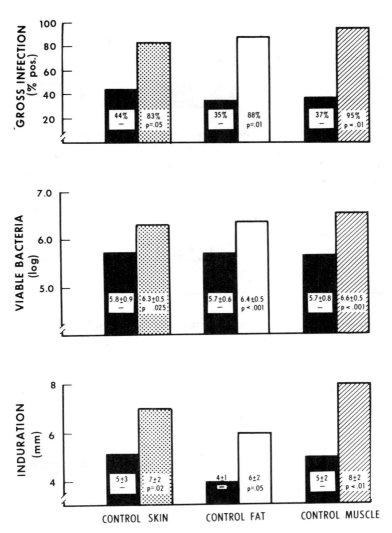

FIG. 1. *Devitalized fat, muscle, and skin potentiated the development of wound infection (S. aureus, 8×10^5).*

The infection potentiating effect of devitalized skin was considerably enhanced by dry thermal injury (Fig. 2). This increased capacity to enhance infection was most apparent in the wounds contaminated with 5×10^4 S. aureus. In these experiments, the incidence of infection (89 percent) in wounds containing dry-burned skin was significantly

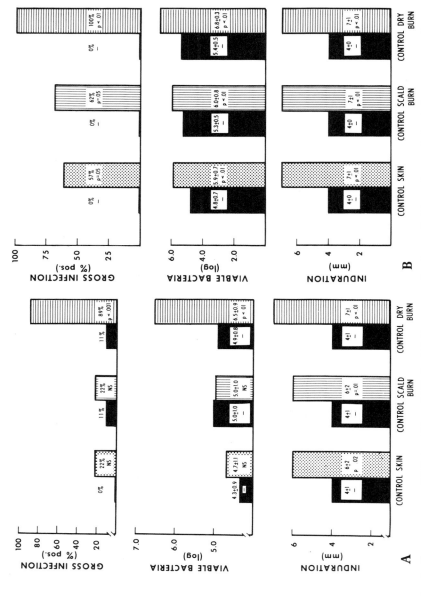

FIG. 2. In the presence of **(A)** 5×10^4 and **(B)** 5×10^5 S. aureus, dry-burned skin enhanced the infection rate of tissues more than either scalded skin or skin not subjected to thermal injury.

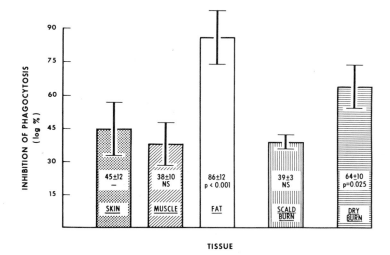

FIG. 3.   *All devitalized tissue inhibited leukocyte bactericidal kill.*

higher than that of wounds subjected to either scald-burned skin (22 percent) or skin without thermal injury (22 percent). The enhanced infection rate of wounds containing dry-burned skin was correlated with an elevated bacterial count and an increased width of its indurated margins.

All devitalized tissue tested *in vivo* inhibited the bactericidal capacity of leukocytes *in vitro* (Fig. 3). In the leukocyte suspensions containing devitalized tissues, the total bacterial count remained significantly higher than in the leukocyte suspensions without devitalized tissue. Devitalized fat and dry-burned skin had the greatest inhibitory effect on leukocyte bacterial kill (Fig. 4).

The damaging effects of fat on leukocyte function was related, in part, to its effect on leukocyte phagocytosis of bacteria. In the presence of devitalized fat, leukocyte phagocytosis was impaired as evidenced by the elevated bacterial count in the supernatant as compared with that in the control leukocyte suspensions. Once ingested, fat appears to limit leukocyte kill. The elevated bacterial counts in the white blood cell sediment exposed to fat were consistent with this view.

Devitalized tissue also supports bacterial growth to a level comparable to that of nutrient broth. Following incubation at 37 C, the growth of bacteria in nutrient broth was similar to that encountered in the presence of devitalized tissue (Fig. 5).

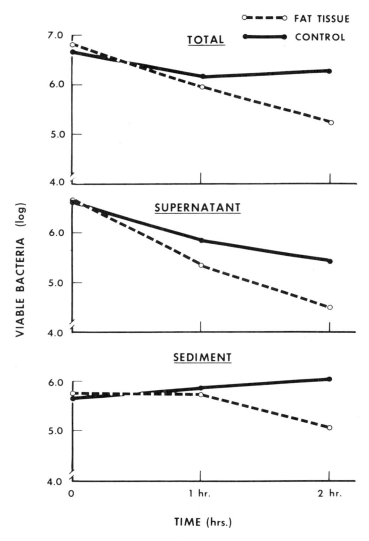

FIG. 4.   In the presence of fat, leukocyte phagocytosis of bacteria as well as kill were impaired.

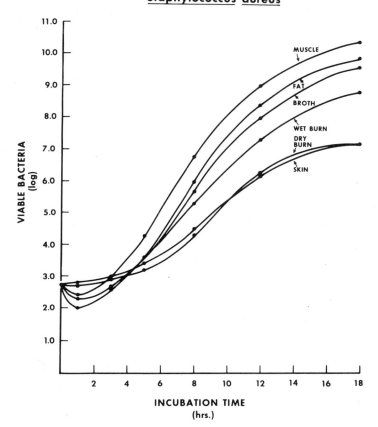

Staphylococcus aureus

FIG. 5.   *Devitalized tissue supports the growth of bacteria to a level comparable to that of nutrient broth.*

SUMMARY

This investigation documents the harmful influences of devitalized tissue on wound defenses and reiterates the importance of wound debridement in the care of the traumatic wound. All of the devitalized soft tissues that were tested damaged the wound's defenses and encouraged the development of infection. The capacity for devitalized fat, muscle, and skin to enhance infection was comparable. The infection-potentiating effect of skin was enhanced by exposing it to a dry thermal injury. This change in the capacity of skin to damage the wound's defenses may be related to the development of a "burn toxin." This experimental finding is consistent with the observation of Algower and Schoenberger[8] who identified a toxin in skin subjected to dry heat. This toxin appears to be generated by the dehydration of a substance naturally occurring in the skin.

The mechanisms by which devitalized soft tissue enhances infection are several. The devitalized tissue acts as a culture medium promoting bacterial growth. In addition, the devitalized tissue inhibits leukocyte phagocytosis of bacteria and subsequent kill. The anaerobic environment within devitalized tissue must also limit leukocyte function (see Chapters 19, 21, and 22). At low oxygen tensions, the killing of certain bacteria by leukocytes is markedly impaired.[9]

While the need for debridement of devitalized tissue is undisputed, identification of the devitalized tissue in wounds remains a challenging problem, especially with muscle. Determination of the viability of muscle is often difficult even for the most experienced surgeon. Some surgeons judge viability of muscle at operation primarily by its contractility; some place greater emphasis on the ability of muscle to bleed; while others judge the condition of muscle by its color and consistency. There is sufficient clinical evidence to show that a muscle is viable if it contracts after being stimulated.[10] Color is of doubtful value in determining the viability of muscle. These clinical indicators of tissue viability are most accurate when the wound is examined 4 to 5 hours after the initial operation. The viability of skin is considerably easier to judge than that of muscle. A sharp line of demarcation is often apparent between the devitalized skin and the viable skin. In skin wounds in which this demarcation is not precise, the distribution of an intravenously injected fluorescein dye within the tissues may prove helpful.[11] Early staining of the injured tissue by fluorescein is evidence of tissue viability.

In some anatomic sites like the trunk, debridement is best accomplished by complete excision of the wound. In these areas, the soft tissue does not contain specialized tissues like nerves or tendons that perform important physical functions. Heavily contaminated serpiginous defects in these regions can be converted into clean wounds by complete excision. The adequacy of debridement may be monitored by forcibly packing the wound with gauze or by coloring the wound surface by a vital dye. Complete excision of the wound that leaves a margin of normal tissue is judged by one's ability to see the gauze or the blue dye during dissection. Suturing the skin edges of the wound prior to excision further minimizes the spread of the wound contaminants into uninjured tissue.

When the wound contains specialized tissues like nerves or tendons, complete excision of the wound is often not feasible. In such cases, high-pressure irrigation followed by excision of all fragments of tissue that are not clearly viable is indicated. In a compound wound of the hand, selective debridement is tedious but essential to remove this dangerous pabulum for bacteria.

A specific exception to the general principle of removing all devitalized tissue is posed by specialized tissues that perform important physical functions, regardless of their viability.[12] Tissues like dura, fascia, and tendon act as free grafts without living cells. Cells from the wound invade the graft as part of the healing process. If these tissues can be rendered surgically clean, they should be left in the wound.

Following debridement, the surgeon's ultimate selection of wound closure technique is dependent on the level of wound contamination and the amount of residual devitalized tissues. In wounds contacted by pus or feces, an infective dose of bacteria will remain in the wound despite the most aggressive wound cleaning. If primary closure of such wounds is attempted, serious infection will usually follow. The development of infection can be prevented by subjecting the wounds to delayed primary closure. As the wound heals, it gains considerable resistance to infection, permitting closure on or after the fifth post-wounding day without subsequent infections.

For high-velocity missile injuries, the magnitude of tissue injury is extensive and difficult to ascertain accurately soon after injury. In these cases, the wound should be explored to remove foreign bodies, to rule out the presence of vascular damage, and to relieve closed compartment pressure when either edema or slow bleeding into a fascia-enclosed muscular compartment is present. The removal of devitalized tissue is advisable but its definition is unclear. Open-wound management is essential with subsequent additional debridement as dictated by the appearance of the wound. When the open wound has gained considerable resistance to infection, on or after the fifth postwounding day, and when the wound contains less than 10^6 bacteria per gram of tissue and is free of devitalized tissue, delayed primary closure is indicated.

Civilian traumatic wounds resulting from impact injuries or low-velocity missiles usually contain devitalized tissue which is easily recognized by the experienced surgeon. Debridement, cleansing, and antibiotic treatment will usually convert these wounds into clean wounds which are amenable to primary closure by either direct approximation of the wound edges or by coverage with a flap or graft with minimal risk of infection.

REFERENCES

1. Jones RC, Shires GT: Principles in the Management of Wounds. In Schwartz SI (ed): Principles of Surgery. New York, McGraw-Hill, 1974
2. Friedrich PL: Die aseptische versorgung frischer wunder, unter mitteilung von theirversuchen uber die auskeimungszeit von infectionserregern in frischer wunden. Arch Klin Chir 57:288, 1898
3. Fildes P: Tetanus VI. The conditions under which tetanus spores germinate in vivo. Br J Exp Pathol 8:387, 1928
4. Altemeier WA, Furste WE: Studies in the virulence of Clostridium welchii. Surgery 25:12, 1949
5. Walker HL and Mason AD Jr: A standard animal model. J Trauma 8:1049, 1968
6. Wickman K: Studies of bacterial interference in experimentally produced burns in guinea pigs. Acta Pathol Microbiol Scand [B] 78:15, 1970
7. Mandel GL. Vest TK: Killing of intraleukocytic Staphylococcus aureus by rifampin: In-viro and in-vivo studies. J Infect Dis 125:486, 1972
8. Allgower M, Cueni LB, Stadtler K, Schoenenberger GA: Burn toxin in mouse skin. J Trauma 13:95, 1973
9. Mandel, GL: Bactericidal activity of aerobic and anaerobic polymorphonuclear neutrophils. Infect Immun 9:337, 1974
10. Scully RE, Artz CP, Sako Y: The criteria for determining the viability of muscle in war wounds. In Studies of the Surgical Research Team Army Medical Service Graduate School, vol. 3, Battle Wounds. Washington.
11. Meyers MB: Prediction and prevention of skin sloughs in radical cancer surgery. Pacific Med Surg 75:315, 1967
12. Peacock EE Jr, Van Winkle W: Repair of skin wounds. In Peacock EE, Van Winkle W (eds): Surgery and Biology of Wound Repair. Philadelphia, Saunders, 1970
13. Mendelson JA, Glover JL: Sphere and shell fragment wounds of soft tissues: An experimental study. J Trauma 7:889, 1967

Comment

The authors have placed a scientific foundation under one of the oldest and most valuable surgical observations—wounds containing dead tissue become infected. Did this need to be done? My answer is yes. First, they tell us a few of the reasons why dead tissue does what it does: (1) it is a good culture medium, (2) it occupies so much attention from leukocytes that they lose their capacity to kill bacteria; (3) as we see in later chapters, the hypoxic white cells in necrotic tissue lose one of their major bacterial killing mechanisms.

If we apply these ideas to a severely ischemic skin flap, we see nothing new in them. On the other hand, let us look at a mastectomy wound or an avulsed but viable perineal skin flap. We did, and we also looked at white cells in the suction drains. They were full of fat!

We compared the bactericidal capacity of leukocytes from blood with fat-laden leukocytes from mastectomy wounds and found that the latter cells did not kill bacteria and, in fact, bacterial growth occurred in their presence.

These data indicate another point at which infection can be prevented—even in apparently clean and viable wounds.

The Physiology of Wound Infection
19

John F. Burke

The increasing number of patients undergoing surgical procedures with a reduced resistance against bacterial invasion adds urgency to efforts being made to understand the basic principles of host defense. It is becoming increasingly clear that the development of surgical therapy will be limited by the inability of the surgeon to restore the patient to a state of normal resistance. The ultimate solution to the problem of postoperative bacterial complications appears to be in a fuller understanding of the processes involved in host resistance, along with the ability to maintain or restore physiological parameters to near normal levels.

The present state of knowledge concerning host resistance against bacterial invasion, although incomplete, provides a starting point for an examination of those avenues which seem likely for future development. The very phrase, "host resistance against bacterial invasion," is all-encompassing. It includes all factors that can be mustered by the organism to defend itself against an invading microorganism. Traditionally, these factors have been divided into the *specific* and the *nonspecific*, depending upon their activity in relation to a single organism. Specific host resistance (or specific immunity) is active against a particular microorganism, depending for the most part on the previous experience of the host with particular microorganisms. Although of great importance in the overall picture of bacterial defenses, it plays a secondary role in preventing postoperative surgical infection. Nonspecific host resistance, on the other hand, is that category of defensive activity that does not depend on the previous experience of the host and is of primary importance in preventing postoperative bacterial problems.

242

The importance of host resistance against bacterial invasion has been neglected. Neither aseptic techniques nor the use of antibiotics has properly recognized that resistance to bacterial invasion depends almost entirely on the efficiency of the host's natural defensive mechanisms. This host resistance cannot, in any measure, be replaced by antibiotic therapy for antibiotic therapy, to be successful in eliminating bacteria from tissue, is dependent on some activity on the part of patients themselves. On the other hand, if tissue resistance against bacterial infection is intact, it provides adequate protection in almost all situations met in daily life. As in other aspects of normal function, however, natural resistance to bacterial invasion varies according to physiological state as well as from tissue to tissue. Periods of decrease in host resistance not only occur with disease, but resistance is also decreased by anesthesia and the surgical procedures themselves. In essence, the concept of normal animal life is dependent on an adequate defense against bacteria.

The extent of protection that normal host resistance provides, as well as the ease with which such resistance can be diluted by abnormal physiology—such as that created by a foreign body—was amply demonstrated in experiments conducted by Elek on human volunteers.[1] In these experiments it was demonstrated that an enormous inoculum of viable staphylococci had to be injected into the dermis of a normal individual before an infection was created. The numbers of bacteria needed to overwhelm the normal host's defensive mechanism were in the millions. Any lesser number of bacteria was effectively dealt with, indicating the efficiency of intact tissue resistance to bacterial infection. A foreign body, however, proved to have an enormous effect on host defenses. If a foreign body in the form of a silk stitch containing approximately 100 viable staphylococci is put in the dermis, a lesion develops which is comparable to the lesion created by millions of organisms. Host defensive forces can easily be blocked. The fate of the primary lodgement of bacteria in tissue—whether or not they persist and develop into an established infection—is determined to a large extent by the defenses of the tissue surrounding the primary lodgement. Further, the issue may be decided in a surprisingly short time; investigations have confirmed the functional importance of early inflammation to the overall defense against bacteria.[2,3] Although the exact sequence of events in early inflammation is far from clear, it is apparent that the first few hours, beginning immediately after the bacterial contamination of the tissue, are of vital importance. Miles has called this time the "decisive period in defense against bacterial invasion."[4] In a series of studies, the effect of blocking a recognized component of early bacterial inflammation and the effect of a modified host resistance on the final size of a developing bacterial lesion were examined.[4] The studies provided information on two points: the contribution the blocked component played in the host's overall ability to control the bacterial invasion, as evidenced by final lesion size, and the point during the development of the bacterial lesion at which the blocked component of host resistance acted to contain the bacteria and, therefore, to determine the size of the mature lesion. The mature lesion was chosen as an end point since a firm relationship exists between mature lesion diameter and the log number of invading bacteria.[5] It is the number of bacteria that survive the rapid initial killing in the tissue that determines the size of the mature lesion.

In experiments in which host resistance was depressed, the expected decrease in bacterial killing and resultant increase in lesion size were observed. An important discovery in the first experiments was that the ability to interrupt the host's normal suppression of a developing lesion was limited to the first few hours following bacterial contamination. In three distinct cases—when the bacteria were injected into the dermis during the time the animal was in shock, in the period of adrenalin ischemia, or closely following injection of the anticomplement substance polyonetholesulfonate (liquoid)—the resulting maximum lesions were substantially larger and more severe than the control lesions. The increase in size and severity of the lesions corresponded to an increase in the number of surviving bacteria. The ability of bacteria to create an inflammatory lesion appeared to be enhanced by the blocking of the host defenses. In addition, it was observed that, although the lesions initiated at the time of, or shortly after, the blocking of a component of the antibacterial defenses were considerably enhanced, lesions that were several hours old before shock or adrenalin ischemia was initiated or before liquoid was injected were not enhanced even though they would not reach a maximum size for an additional 20 (or more) hours. At 24 hours these lesions were the same size as controls.

Three concepts emerge from these experiments. First, certain tissue antibacterial mechanisms that are inhibited by a reduced or absent local blood flow or by anticomplementary substances allow bacterial survival in the tissue in unusual proportions, resulting in a considerably enlarged area of tissue damage. Second, these particular antibacterial mechanisms exert their effect in controlling the lesion within the first 3 hours following tissue contamination. Third, it is during this short, early period that the ultimate size of the lesion is determined. Thus, in the normal state, tissue defenses appear to act immediately over a very short period of time. If, as was done in laboratory experiments, defenses are made inoperative before the contaminating bacteria are killed, the bacteria are allowed to multiply, resulting in an increased area of tissue damage and a larger mature lesion.

This short period, which is decisive, is the time during which the inhibition of certain defense mechanisms results in lesion enhancement. The importance of understanding the existence of this "decisive period" is greatest with respect to determining the means for increasing host resistance through the use of exogenous substances such as antibiotics, which could add to the host's natural abilities. As a corollary to understanding of the decisive period, the time of maximum enhancement was found when the tissue defenses were inhibited maximally—that is, inhibited immediately before or at the same time that the tissue was contaminated with bacteria. Thus, susceptibility to enhancement steadily declined to the end of the decisive period when the lesion could not be enhanced at all. An example of this development is shown in Figure 1, which demonstrates the effect of local adrenalin ischemia on the ability of the dermis to control a standard inoculum of viable staphylococci.

The premise that there is a period of intense, highly effective host antibacterial activity, beginning immediately on arrival of bacteria in tissue, which contains the bacterial invasion in less than 4 hours, suggests that there is value in examining the possibility of enhancing host defenses during this decisive period. The implications for clinical medicine are great, particularly for surgery, in which infection following operations may severely complicate the patient's recovery. Theoretically, antibiotic substances could augment the natural mechanisms of bacterial resistance in tissue. In most cases, their bacteriocidal or bacteriostatic activity does not perceptibly interfere with nat-

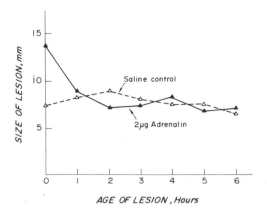

FIG. 1.   Adrenalin ischemia greatly enhances infectability. This is demonstrated by the lesion size which results when ischemia is produced within the first hour or two of injection of bacteria (see Fig. 2).

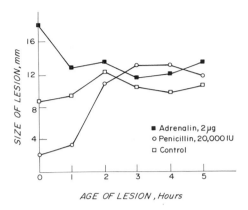

FIG. 2. The decisive period demonstrated by the adrenalin curve is compared with the effective period of antibiotics as demonstrated by the penicillin curve.

ural host mechanisms but affects bacteria directly. The two forces, natural host resistance and antibiotics, should actually be additive or, ideally, synergistic in preventing or reducing the size of final bacterial lesions. In experimental[6] and clinical[7-10] studies, this has, in fact, proven to be the case. There is a period during which it is possible to augment the host's antibacterial mechanisms by the use of an antibiotic. This "effective period of a preventive antibiotic" occurs when its antibacterial activity is coordinated with that of the host to produce more effective bacterial killing and a smaller lesion. This is the opposite effect from that seen using an agent to block host resistance during the decisive period. Figure 2 compares the *decisive period*, demonstrated by adrenalin ischemia, with the *effective period*, demonstrated by the effect of penicillin on an experimental staphylococcal lesion. The same biologic characteristics are involved in both cases. If penicillin is given at the same time the wound is contaminated, the resulting lesion is similar to a lesion produced by an autoclaved (i.e., killed) bacterial suspension. If, on the other hand, tissue is contaminated and penicillin is not administered until 3 hours after bacterial contamination, the lesion is similar to the infection seen in an animal given no penicillin but contaminated with a staphylococcal suspension. Experiments designed to gather data on the blocking of the host mechanism and to determine the decisive period for action reveal three major points. First, nonspecific host resistance against bacterial invasion is a composite of a number of distinct factors, some of which operate locally at the site of the bacterial contamination. Second, the interaction between host forces and bacteria begins at the moment bacteria arrive in the tissue; there is no "grace period." Third, host defenses have shown a period of intense, effective activity beginning at the moment of contamination and ending within the first few hours following the arrival of bacteria, even though the lesion continues to develop in the sense of a classic inflammation for an additional 20 hours or more. This means that a number of important components of patients' ability to defend themselves against bacterial invasion exert their effect for a surprisingly short interval. Growth of bacteria and the development of the bacterial lesion itself appear to provide some protection for the bacteria within the lesion.

If this knowledge is applied to the clinical situation, it is clear that considerable attention must be paid to the moment at which contamination of the tissue takes place—the moment when the host's defensive mechanisms, if functioning, are most effective. Their capacities decrease for the next few hours, and the struggle to prevent infection appears to be decided early. This information may be used clinically in surgery in appropriate patients, thus reducing the risk of postoperative sepsis.[11,12]

REFERENCES

1. Elek SD: Experimental staphylococcal infections in the skin of man. Ann NY Acad Sci 65:85, 1956
2. Miles AA, Miles EM, Burke JF: The value and duration of defense reactions of the skin to the primary lodgement of bacteria. Brit J Exp Pathol 38:79, 1957
3. Burke JF, Miles AA: The sequence of vascular events in early infectious inflammation. J Pathol Bacteriol 76:1, 1958
4. Miles AA: Nonspecific defense reactions in bacterial infections. Ann NY Acad Sci 66:356, 1956
5. Miles AA, Niven J: The enhancement of infection during shock produced by bacterial toxins and other agents. Brit J Exp Pathol 31:73, 1950
6. Burke JF: The effective period of preventive antibiotic action in experimental incisions and dermal lesions. Surgery 50:161, 184, 1961
7. Boyd RJ, Burke JF, Colton T: A double blind clinical trial of prophylactic antibiotics in hip fracture patients. J Bone Joint Surg 55A:1251, 1973
8. Polk HC Jr, Lopez-Mayor JF: Postoperative wound infection. Surgery 66:97, 1969
9. Bernard HR, Cole WR: The prophylaxis of surgical infection: The effect of prophylactic antimicrobial drugs on the incidence of infection following potentially contaminated operations. Surgery 56:151, 1964
10. Nelson RM, Henson CB, Peterson CA, et al: Effective use of prophylactic antibiotics in open heart surgery. Arch Surg 90:731, 1965
11. Burke JF: Preventive antibiotic management in surgery. Ann Rev Med 24:289, 1973
12. Ballinger WF, Collins JA, Drucker WR, et al: Manual on Control of Infection in Surgical Patients. Saunders, Philadelphia, 1975

Comment

To Dr. Burke and Professor A. A. Miles goes the credit for the discovery of the critical and determinative periods after innoculation of bacteria in tissue. This is an immensely powerful concept and provides an important key to the economic, safe, and effective use of preventive antibiotics in surgery.

I have a little trouble extrapolating the *exact timing* of the critical period of an innoculum of bacteria injected into normal tissue to the situation in which a small innoculum is allowed to contaminate a wound. In the experiments reported here, the lesions were fully developed in 20 hours, whereas wound infections characteristically appear in 5 to 7 days. Some wound infections are delayed for months or even years. Therefore, it is difficult for me to accept the conclusion that one might be tempted to draw from these data—that *everything* one can accomplish in terms of preventing infection is accomplished by the end of the third hour after the wound is closed. It seems obvious that the first few hours are terribly important, but perhaps they are not all-important. Dr. Burke has not made this claim, and one should be careful not to assume it. It seems well demonstrated, however, that about everything one is likely to accomplish *with antibiotics* will be accomplished in the first few postoperative hours. Jennings et al. (1977) have shown in experimental incision in rats with a distant, active infection that the "critical period" remains just as Dr. Burke has described it for injected bacteria.

These concepts have allowed us to construct an appealing policy for the use of preventive antibiotics at the University of California, San Francisco. We base this policy on a classification which Dr. Edlich also has helped define. Wounds are classified into four categories: clean wounds (in which the innoculum is less than 10^4 bacteria), clean-contaminated wounds (in which the innoculum is less than 10^6 bacteria), heavily contaminated wounds, and wounds contacted by pus or infected fluid in which the contamination is roughly 10^8/cc of contaminating substance. The classification scheme and the preventive antibiotic policy are reproduced for those who would be interested in using them (pages 250–53).

To Dr. Burke belongs much of the credit for our new ability to limit preventive antibiotics, because his research has allowed surgeons to put a time limit to the use of preventive antibiotics. (A further practical discussion between surgeons experienced in this field can be found in Hunt et al. 1975.)

Dr. Burke has placed antibiotics in the role of aiding host defenses. "Host defenses" is an easy general concept, but its details have been elusive. The chapters by Hohn (21) and Hunt et al. (22) demonstrate many of the details. One will note that there are ways of bolstering host defenses other than with antibiotics. Unfortunately, none are as easily used or as readily accessible. The important aspect of this chapter is that it provides the basic facts needed to use antibiotics effectively with minimal effect on hospital or patient ecology and with minimal expense.

REFERENCES

Jennings SA, Robson MC, and Jennings MM: Preventing wound infection from distant endogenous sources in the rat. J Surg Res 22:16, 1977

Hunt TK, Alexander JW, Burke JF, MacLean LD: Antibiotics in surgery. Arch Surg 110:148, 1975

Proposal for the Use of Preventive
Antibiotics in Surgery

The following is a proposal for unified indications for the use of preventive antibiotics in surgery. It represents a consensus among surgeons and makes the following basic assumptions:

1. Antibiotics are effective antimicrobials even when given before infection is apparent. The probability of effective use is based on the statistical chance of matching the contaminating organisms with an effective antibiotic(s). Unfortunately, attempting to increase the spectrum of preventive antibiotics with combinations of agents is prohibitively expensive in terms of drug reactions and interactions and emergence of resistant strains.
2. Antibiotics rapidly enter tissue (defined as that portion of the body outside the lymphovascular system). Based on studies in humans and animals, full equilibration of antibiotic between the vascular system and the tissue is achieved within 90 minutes in an area of damaged vasculature. Tissues without damaged vasculature equilibrate more rapidly.
3. In animal tests and by inference from human tests, the chance of most effective prevention of infection is highest when there is a one-time contamination (the operation) which occurs when the antibiotic(s) is already at an effective concentration in the blood and tissues. The chance of effective use is lost by about 3 hours after the operative wound is closed.
4. Numerous studies in humans prove that, in operations with random contamination, the effectiveness of prophylaxis is small to nil.
5. The frequency of significant adverse reaction to antibiotics in the individual patient is estimated at about 5 percent. It seems clear that to use antibiotics to decrease the likelihood of trivial infection or that due to random contamination is to (often) accept a risk greater than that of the infection itself.
6. Each use of antibiotics extends the chance for resistant bacterial strains to develop in the hospital ecology. Each unnecessary use of antibiotics thus endangers not only the patient receiving it but many other patients (both present and future) as well. It is, therefore, the responsibility of each surgeon using preventive antibiotics to re-

strict their use to only those patients who can be expected to benefit and to use the minimal amount of antibiotic necessary to accomplish that benefit. The protocol presented below is intended to assist in making these judgments.

The following protocol is submitted:

1. Preventive antibiotics are best begun at the first sign of more than random contamination. When the use of preventive antibiotic is predictable, the therapy should be started slightly before operation is begun, or very early in its course. There is no need to give an antibiotic more than 2 hours prior to operation except for operations that will traverse tissue which is or has been infected.
2. If antibiotics are not given until the operation has begun, there is an advantage to giving the antibiotic in bolus dose intravenously. (Potential respiratory depressants, such as kanamycin or gentamycin, or polymyxins should *not* be given in bolus.)
3. For *clean* operations (see classification below) in which a foreign body is not deliberately implanted, prophylactic antibiotics will have little or no use since the expected infection rate is well below 5 percent. Operations classified as *clean-contaminated* or *lightly contaminated* would not ordinarily justify routine preoperative antibiotics since the expected infection rate without antibiotics is less than 5 percent. They might, by the surgeon's judgment, however, qualify at a higher infection probability if more than the usual contamination is encountered during the procedure. Operations classified as *heavily contaminated* have been followed by infection rates greater than 5 percent when antibiotics were not used. Therefore, they ordinarily qualify for the use of prophylactic antibiotics unless the consequences of infection are trivial enough to totally obviate the need for antibiotics, e.g., hemorrhoid resections or minor urological surgery. Assessment of the patient's resistance or infection risk may affect the decision; that is, an immune-suppressed or neutropenic patient is more likely to become infected in a clean-contaminated operative site than a normal patient.
4. For operations in which foreign body is not implanted, prophylactic antibiotics should be stopped within 3 to 24 hours after operation.
5. Operations in which a vitally important foreign body, such as arterial grafting, heart valve replacement, or joint replacement, is implanted may qualify for preventive antibiotics in the surgeon's judgment. After such use, preventive antibiotics should be withdrawn within 48 hours after surgery or within 24 hours of the time that intravascular tubes are withdrawn. The major single exception to

this rule would be in patients who have undergone previous operation in which the operative site became infected or in whom cultures of tissues from the operative area show the presence of significant numbers of pathogenic organisms. In this case, the antibiotic chosen for continuing treatment should be selected on the basis of sensitivities of the previously infecting organism. We cannot make a firm recommendation on the duration of therapy in this instance.

Operative Wound Classification According to Contamination/Infection Risk

Class 1: Clean

Nontraumatic; no inflammation encountered; no break in sterile technique; respiratory, alimentary, genitourinary tracts not entered

Reported infection rates are usually 1 to 4 percent. In general, no antibiotics are needed unless the host defenses are suppressed or unless the consequences of infection are catastrophic—heart valve replacement, etc. Drains are not used unless blood or fluid must be evacuated.

Class 2: Clean-Contaminated

Gastrointestinal or respiratory tracts entered without significant spillage; appendectomy not perforated, no cloudy peritoneal exudate; prepared oropharynx or vagina entered; genitourinary or biliary tracts entered in absence of infected urine or bile; minor break in sterile technique

Reported infection rates are 5 to 15 percent. Here the surgeon must use his judgment about using preoperative antibiotics. It should not be necessary to use antibiotics in most cases of biliary or small intestinal surgery unless host defenses are suppressed. When consequences of infection are trivial (anal and minor mouth procedures), do not use antibiotics. Delayed primary closure may be considered.

Class 3: Contaminated

Major break in sterile technique; gross spillage from gastrointestinal tract; traumatic fresh, wound; entrance of genitourinary or biliary tracts in presence of infected urine or bile; colon entered with any spill of content

Reported infection rates are about 16 to 25 percent, although many centers are reporting less with preventive antibiotics. In this category, most patients will need antibiotic supplementation unless the operation is trivial, as in anal surgery. Delayed primary or secondary closure techniques should be used frequently.

Class 4: Dirty and infected

Acute bacterial inflammation or pus encountered; transection of

Infection rates mean little here but are often over 25 percent. Here, either de-

Class 4 (cont.)

"clean" tissue for the purpose of surgical access to a collection of pus; perforated viscus encountered; traumatic wound with retained devitalized tissue, foreign bodies, fecal contamination and/ or delayed treatment, or from dirty source

layed closure of skin and subcutaneous tissues or antibiotics or both should be used. Antibiotics are not usually necessary for drainage of a small abscess.

Modified from Altemeier WA et al. (eds): Manual on Control of Infection in Surgical Patients. Philadelphia, Lippincott, 1976

Environmental Control of Microbial Contamination in the Operating Room
20

Morris L.V. French, Harold E. Eitzen,
Merrill A. Ritter, and Diane S. Leland

Infection control in the operating room involves a combination of many factors, including the health status or resistance level to infection of the surgical patient, the type of surgery involved, surgical technique, and the extent and type of endogenous and environmental contamination which finds its way to the surgical wound.

We have attempted to evaluate the importance of environmental contamination in the surgical suite with respect to surgical wound infection. Our studies have been performed by a team interested in infection control in surgery which was composed of an orthopedic surgeon, a microbiologist, an epidemiologist and an engineer. Together, this team has analyzed the importance of a wide variety of factors that have real or potential importance in the control of surgical infection. It was the intention of the team to evaluate the relative importance of the many factors involved in surgery and then to rate their relative importance in order to establish "high-priority" factors. Finally, the team has attempted to study alternate methods or procedures to replace or remove factors that have been determined to be important in the control of infections.

METHODS

In attempting to evaluate various sources of contamination in the operating room, we have developed several simple, reproducible microbial sampling methods.[1-7] These methods may be used to assess contamination of surfaces, air, instruments, surgical team members, and the patient. We do not recommend routine sampling; but, for research purposes or for investigation of specific problems, we recommend the following techniques.

Air

Air sampling in the operating room should measure microbial fallout rather than air-suspended microbes. Types and numbers of bacteria falling into the wound and on instruments is of primary importance. Therefore, the sampling sites must be in the clean operating zone. Such sampling can be accomplished by using sterile agar plates prepared as follows: Wrap 150 mm glass petri dishes in the same material that is used for wrapping surgical instruments. Sterilize and dry the dishes. Then unwrap the dishes in a laminar air flow hood and fill them with sterile 5 percent sheep blood agar. Rewrap the plates and test them for sterility by incubating them at 37 C for 24 hours. The plate is inspected for contamination when it is unwrapped.

One sterile plate is placed on the instrument table and another next to the wound site. The wound site can be held in place with a portion of sterile adhesive drape. The time is recorded when the cover is removed and again when it is closed. The results of settle plate sampling are expressed in colony forming units (CFU)/sq ft/hr by using the following formula for the 150 mm petri dishes:

$$\text{CFU/sq ft/hr} = \frac{\text{CFU}}{0.16499 \text{ sq ft} \div t(\text{hr})}$$

Instruments

Large-mouth canning jars filled with nutrient broth or thioglycollate broth are useful for sterility testing of large items such as hemostats, forceps, and sponges. Items to be tested are placed into the jars with sterile instruments rather than gloved hands. Gloved hands may be contaminated after a few minutes of surgery.

Surfaces

The Rodac plate (4 inches square) filled with 5 percent sheep blood agar is suggested for surface sampling. This combination simplifies the tasks of enumeration and identification of organisms. The Rodac plate is recommended rather than the traditional cotton swab technique because the surface of the Rodac plate is delineated.

Appropriate neutralizers must be included in the media utilized when one is sampling surfaces containing either antiseptics or disinfectants. Dey-Engle agar contains neutralizers for most antiseptics and disinfectants. However, many active ingredients of antiseptic and disinfectant compounds are effectively neutralized by the protein found in 5 percent sheep blood agar.

Personnel and Patients

Patients and personnel may be sampled if they are suspected of being the source of a particular organism such as *Staphylococcus aureus*. A specimen collected from the anterior nares is satisfactory for this type of analysis. A sterile cotton swab moistened in nutrient broth or saline should be used for collecting the specimen.

DISCUSSION

Air

In conventional operating rooms, the air is prefiltered with either an electrostatic precipitator or a bag filtration unit. Each of these devices reduces the microbial content of air by 86 to 94 percent. The air is then humidified to about 50 percent relative humidity, and the temperature is adjusted to approximately 70°F. The air, prior to entering the operating room, passes through high-efficiency filters (99.99 percent). The number of air changes per hour is usually 10 to 15 compared with approximately six air changes per hour in a family dwelling.

The fallout rate of the air in most empty operating rooms is less than 10 CFU/sq ft/hr. Operating rooms that have been cleaned and left idle overnight show very few bacteria when they are tested the following morning. If the same operating room is measured for microbial fallout during surgery when it contains six to nine surgical team members and a patient, the average microbial fallout rises to approximately 300 CFU/sq ft/hr.[8]

The microbial fallout is highest at the wound site and instrument table, and the lowest fallout rate is at the periphery of the room. With a fallout rate of about 300 CFU/sq ft/hr and with a surgical clean zone surface area of approximately 25 sq ft, 7500 bacteria will settle onto the clean zone during a one-hour operation. Most operations, however, last longer than one hour. The microorganisms falling onto the surface of the clean zone contaminate not only the open wound, but all of the instruments as well. All instruments will show contamination within a 2-hour period. We have also found that gloves become contaminated rapidly at the beginning of the procedure. It has been shown by several investigators that personnel shed approximately 10,000 bacteria per minute, though many of these microorganisms die quickly because of environmental trauma. From the information presented here it is obvious that the value of proper instrument sterilization and of careful aseptic technique can be rapidly negated by high levels of microbial fallout.

There are some ways that this microbial contamination can be reduced. Ultraviolet light is effective, but not practical. In the last few years laminar air flow has been suggested as a means of controlling airborne contamination. By using environmental control, of which the laminar air flow system is a part, infection rates have been reduced (in uncontrolled studies) from over 6 percent to as low as 0.4 percent. Laminar air flow reduced microbial contamination from 300 to less than 20 CFU/sq ft/hr. The equipment costs approximately $20,000 for the average operating room.

Instruments

Instruments to be used for surgery are normally unwrapped from their packages and placed on instrument tables. This practice allows the instruments to be exposed to microbial fallout prior to and during the entire surgical procedure. We have defined appropriate sequential sets of instruments to be used for each type of surgical procedure. Instruments are placed into pans according to the order of their use during the surgical procedure; for example, five trays of instruments have been established for a total hip replacement. These wrapped trays are left unopened until the time of their use, thereby reducing exposure to microbial fallout in the procedure. Used instruments are removed from the clean zone before wound closure. A new set of instruments and gloves are employed at this time so that the irrigated wound is closed in the cleanest possible state.

Theater Surfaces

The surfaces of most operating rooms consist of nonporous material which is easily cleaned. With respect to surfaces, the greatest hazard in the operating room is the accumulation of dust and lint, both of which may contain fungi. There are few horizontal surfaces in the operating room, but those that do exist, such as the operating room lamp, must be carefully cleaned to insure that they are free of dust and lint. The walls and floor must be free of obvious soil. It should be remembered that the most important site in the operating room is the wound site and that microorganisms on the floor and the wall do not have easy access into the wound. These surfaces should be cleaned with soap or detergents which contain some type of disinfectant to reduce microbial buildup.

Personnel and Patients

SURGICAL ATTIRE.   Present-day surgical garments do not effectively contain microorganisms being shed by the surgical team. Our studies have shown that plastic gowns reduce surface contamination by 71.8 percent when compared with paper material.[9] Paper gowns showed 33 percent less contamination than cloth. Although the plastic gowns controlled contamination, they were extremely uncomfortable. More research is needed to develop a gown that is comfortable, yet capable of containing microorganisms being shed by the surgical team.

The data collected on in-use face mask studies indicates that face masks have little effect on microbial contamination in the operating room.[10] The major purpose of face masks in surgery is to protect the wound from droplets of saliva expelled by the team members when talking.

No statistical difference in microbial fallout was found when caps, cloth hoods, and no head cover were compared. A hooded gown that is comfortable, but impervious to moisture and microbial migration, is needed.

Gloves become contaminated very quickly probably from heavy microbial fallout. Our studies indicate that flaws or holes in gloves do not increase surface contamination.[6] Cruse reports that holes in gloves do not influence surgical wound infection rates.[11] Since gloves do become contaminated, it is suggested that new gloves be put on when instrument trays are changed and just prior to closure of the properly irrigated, ready-to-close wound.

ANTISEPTICS.   Contamination of the surgical clean zone with indigenous skin flora organisms from personnel or patient is an obvious hazard. Therefore, a thorough antiseptic cleansing of the hands and arms of surgical personnel as well as cleansing of the patient's surgical site have been an important aspect of presurgery preparation for many years. We have attempted to assess the importance of contamination that is of "skin flora" origin. We have found only minimal amounts of bacteria on antiseptic-scrubbed skin and do not believe this to be a significant source of surgical wound infection.

While in the process of comparing the contamination present on hands and at the surgical site, we have also been able to evaluate the antiseptics available today. All of the antiseptic products tested for efficacy in degerming hands or the surgical skin site were found to be effective, and there was not a statistically significant difference between them. In our opinion, surgical team members may choose a degerming agent on the basis of personal preference or cost.

From 1975 to the present we have utilized a poloxamer-iodine compound to degerm the wound site at the time of surgery. No preliminary wound site scrubbing was performed either at the time of surgery or during the previous night. Using the disinfecting agents and procedures just described and operating in a horizontal, unidirectional laminar flow surgical suite, we have maintained and documented an infection rate of 0.47 percent in 633 total joint arthroplasties (423 hips, 210 knees).

WOUND DRAPES. At Indiana University Medical Center, an evaluation of adhesive plastic drapes and of cloth surgical drapes was made.[12] These studies were done both during surgery and in the laboratory. The plastic drape prevents bacterial penetration and lateral migration, eliminates multiplication of skin bacteria under the drape within the time studied, and aids in holding cloth drapes in place. Cloth drapes, especially when wet, were penetrated easily by bacteria. Lateral migration under cloth drapes was not possible to assess because of the high level of penetration.

The effect of the drape type on wound contamination was studied. Deep wound cultures collected just prior to wound closure showed 60 percent wound contamination when a cloth drape was used and only 6 percent contamination when a plastic drape was employed. In addition to the positive aseptic benefits afforded by plastic adhesive drapes, esthetic features, such as a more delineated operating field and elimination of towel clips, make this product a useful adjunct to the surgeon's armamentarium.

Cruse reported that plastic adhesive drapes do not reduce or increase surgical wound infection.[11] We suspect, however, that heavy microbial fallout onto the surgical clean zone and its contents may make it impossible to determine the effect that drapes, gloves, and so on have on infection rates. We find it difficult to believe that cloth drapes soaked with body and irrigating fluids do not affect wound contamination.

CONCLUSIONS

Analysis of the factors important in infection control in surgery is extremely difficult because there are so many. We have attempted to reduce or limit the number of variables by limiting our studies to relatively healthy patients requiring clean surgical procedures. Within these limitations, we believe a few important conclusions can be made.

Procedures normally used in preparing for and performing surgery are excellent. The methods used for sterilization of instruments, materials, and surgical garments are effective and dependable. Normal aseptic technique, as used by the surgical teams we have observed and studied, is excellent. Surgical hand scrubs, surgical site preparative agents, and surgical gloves currently used are effective.

One significant factor which has been neglected is the microbial shedding from surgical team members. This shedding produces significant airborne contamination which results in the contamination of sterile instruments, gloved hands, and surgical wounds. Conventional cotton surgical garments used by most surgical teams are not effective in controlling microbial shedding.

A variety of techniques or procedures has been utilized in attempting to control shedding and airborne contamination. Limiting the number of individuals in the operating room and reducing activity in the room prior to surgery have not been effective in reducing airborne contamination. The use of the laminar air flow system is one of the more effective methods. In our opinion, microbial fallout and airborne contamination can be further controlled by the development and use of surgical garments that are comfortable yet effective in controlling microbial shedding.

Finally, we feel that it is important for surgeons to be aware of their clean wound infection rate. We feel that it is within the capability of today's surgical teams to obtain clean wound infection rates of 0.5 to 1.0 percent by directing appropriate attention to the last significant source of contamination—microbial shedding.

REFERENCES

1. French MLV, Ritter MA, Eitzen HE, Hart JB: Microbial evaluation of reusable and disposable laparotomy sponges. Surg Gynecol Obstet 137:465, 1973
2. French MLV, Ritter MA, Hart JB: A new approach for microbiological sampling in the comparison of a clean room versus a conventional room during actual surgery. Ber Int Symp Reinraumtech 19:72, 1973.
3. French MLV, Ritter MA, Hart JB, Eitzen HE: Clean air symposium—Part II: A systems analysis approach to postoperative wound infections—Phase II. Cleve Clin Q 40:221, 1973
4. Hart JB, French MLV, Eitzen HE, Ritter MA: Rodac plate-holding device for sampling surfaces during surgery. Appl Microbiol 26:417, 1973
5. Ritter MA, French MLV, Eitzen HE: Bacterial contamination of the surgical knife. Clin Orthop 108:158, 1975
6. Ritter MA, French MLV, Eitzen HE: Evaluation of microbial contamination of surgical gloves during actual use. Clin Orthop 117:303, 1976

7. Ritter MA, French MLV, Hart, JB: Microbiological studies in a horizontal wall-less laminar air-flow operating room during actual surgery. Clin Orthop 97:16, 1973

8. French MLV, Eitzen HE, Ritter MA: Increasing evidence for controlling microbial contamination in the operating room. In International Symposium on Contamination Control Proceedings, London, Black, 1974

9. Alford DJ, Ritter MA, French MLV, Hart JB: The operating room gown as a barrier to bacterial shedding. Am J Surg 125:589, 1973

10. Ritter MA, Eitzen HE, French MLV, Hart JB: The operating room environment as affected by people and the surgical face mask. Clin Orthop 111:147, 1975

11. Cruse PJE, Foord R: A five-year prospective study of 23,649 surgical wounds. Arch Surg 107:206, 1973

12. French MLV, Eitzen HE, Ritter, MA: The plastic surgical adhesive drape. Ann Surg 184:46, 1976

Comment

The authors have contributed a "state of the art" essay on cleanliness in the operating suite. In remarkably few words, they summarize their methods of measuring exogenous contamination and their results, and draw basic conclusions about the current practice of aseptic technique.

There is no question that the surgical team itself is the weakness of the current system of asepsis. The patient's resistance, as modified by the surgeon and anesthesiologist, is the other major weakness in the scheme of infection control.

Two other techniques probably deserve mention here, though they are a little out of the purview of the paper. The first is the quantitative sampling of bacteria from the wound by means of swabs or precisely measured squares of fabric velour (Rahaave 1974). The second is the use of a nonadherent plastic wound protector drape to isolate the wound (only) from contamination.

The significance of the first technique is that the quantitative assay of surface bacteria on the freshly cut wound correlates with wound infection though it does not correlate well with burn-wound infection. The use of an established human infection is an expensive end-point in a clinical study. It is rare enough that its use demands huge, expensive, time-consuming studies to test even the simplest concepts. It is dangerous enough to lay serious question on the ethics of eliminating even improved (but commonly used) anti-infection techniques as a study object or mechanism by which controlled trials can be designed. I hope that the quantitative assessment of contamination at the wound will replace established human wound infection as a means of determining the effectiveness (cost or otherwise) of both new and old aseptic techniques.

The significance of the second development, the wound protector, is that it shields what is usually the most vulnerable operative area, the wound, from contamination during most of any surgical procedure which enters a body cavity. One clinical study (of which the end point was wound infection) attests to its effectiveness. Another does not. Rahaave's study used quantitative wound culture as noted above and attests to its value. A similar study ongoing in our laboratory also attests to its effectiveness. Using wound isolation as a principle may initiate the problem of contamination by the surgical team. It also has the obvious advantage of protection from bacteria derived from the patient. Aseptic technique has an end point which is well short of elimination of all bacteria from the operative site. It should be pursued to its logical ends—it seems that it *must* be pursued. No matter how effective it is, however, asepsis can never excuse surgeons from perfecting their surgical techniques or from their responsibility to support host defenses.

REFERENCE

Rahaave D: Aseptic barriers of plastic to prevent bacterial contamination in operation wounds. Acta Chir Scand 140:585, 1974

Host Resistance to Infection: Established and Emerging Concepts

21

David C. Hohn

The humoral and cellular immune systems as well as phagocytic leukocytes have long been known to be the major components in mammalian resistance to infection. Detailed knowledge of the molecular mechanisms of microbial containment and destruction, however, has emerged only recently. Elucidation of these defense mechanisms has begun to indicate why healthy, well-perfused tissues have substantial natural resistance to infection while resistance to infection in poorly perfused and/or traumatized tissues may be low. With improved methods of quantitative assessment of various host defense functions has come the identification of acquired immune disorders in surgical patients, and the development of methods for preserving or augmenting resistance to infection appears imminent.

In most bacterial and fungal infections, the killing and destruction of microbes is accomplished by the phagocytic leukocytes and macrophages. In most surgical infections, phagocytic leukocytes are initially the most important elements in the host defense system. This chapter reviews the major established concepts in the areas of phagocytosis and microbial killing and then will examine certain emerging concepts which have contributed to our understanding of the factors responsible for "natural" resistance to infection in surgical wounds.

CHEMOTAXIS AND OPSONIZATION

After bacterial contamination has occurred, neutrophils and then monocytes migrate from capillaries to the locus of developing infection;

this process is called *chemotaxis*. The critical elements are (1) a contractile protein system within the leukocyte which provides the motility, (2) receptors at the cell membrane that "recognize" certain chemotactic factors and direct cell motion toward areas where these factors are most concentrated, and (3) a source of chemotactic substances. A variety of substances derived from bacteria, from injured tissues, and from the complement system exhibit chemotactic activity for neutrophils and monocytes.[1] It now appears that the most important complement-derived chemotactic substances are C3a and C5a which are proteolytic fragments of complement factors C3 and C5.[2] As is shown in Figure 1, the activation of C3 and C5 can proceed either via the classical hemolytic complement sequence (C1,2,4) which is triggered by microbial attachment of specific antibody, or by the alternate properdin pathway which may be directly activated by bacteria in the absence of antibody. In either case chemotactic fragments are liberated and diffuse into tissues attracting phagocytes to the area. C5a and C3a are also "anaphylatoxic," causing increased vascular permeability, histamine release from mast cells, and contraction of smooth muscle both *in vitro* and *in vivo*.[3] Recently, the amino acid sequence of C5a has been determined; it was found that anaphylactic activity is conferred by an arginine residue at the C-terminal end of the molecule.[4] Removal of this arginine abolishes anaphylatoxic activity while chemotactic activity is preserved.

After the neutrophils are attracted to the nidus, recognition and ingestion of the offending organisms must occur. These steps are facilitated by humorally derived factors, termed *opsonins*, which bind to the microbial surface and interact with receptors on the leukocyte

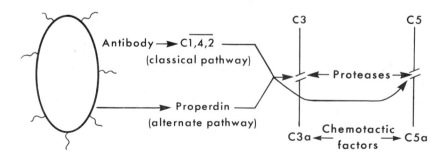

FIG. 1.   *Interaction between bacteria and serum causes cleavage of C3 and C5, and production of chemotactic factors C3a and C5a. This cleavage is accomplished by either the classical antibody-activated, hemolytic complement pathway, or by the antibody-independent alternate properdin pathway.*

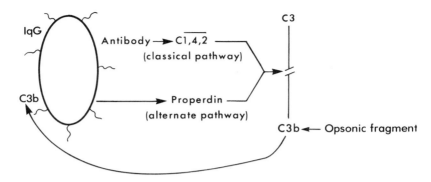

FIG. 2.   *Opsonization of bacteria is required for efficient phagocytosis of most microorganisms. The major opsonic component is a proteolytic fragment of C3 which is produced either through activation of the classical hemolytic pathway or the alternate properdin pathway. This fragment, C3b, binds to the microbial surface and interacts with receptors on the phagocyte membrane to promote phagocytosis.*

to accelerate the rate of ingestion. As shown in simplified form in Figure 2, one of the major opsonic substances is a proteolytic fragment of C3 called C3b. Like that of C3a and C5a, the formation of C3b can also be initiated via either the alternate or the classical complement pathway.

A number of clinical disorders have been recognized in which defective chemotaxis and opsonization are associated with an increased susceptibility to infection. Of particular interest to surgeons are findings of depressed chemotaxis in patients with major traumatic and burn injuries and in patients with malnutrition.[5,6,7] Alexander recently has suggested that overwhelming sepsis may cause consumption of available opsonins and lead to a self-perpetuating, consumptive opsonin deficiency.[8] Another opsonic factor, α_2-surface glycoprotein, closely resembles cold-insoluble globulin and is essential for effective clearance of organisms by the reticuloendothelial system. Saba and associates[9] have recently documented a deficiency of α_2-surface binding glycoprotein in septic surgical and trauma patients and have shown that the administration of cryoprecipitate caused restoration of opsonic function with apparent clinical recovery. Depletion of complement factors has been convincingly demonstrated in certain serious viral diseases, in cryptococcal sepsis, and during surgical procedures.[10,11] If such findings are confirmed, opsonin repletion may be a new modality for augmenting host defenses in the treatment of sepsis.

INGESTION

After the phagocytes have been attracted to the site of contamination and after the bacteria have been coated with opsonic proteins, the opsonized bacteria attach to surface receptors on the leukocyte, triggering the ingestion process. As shown in Figure 3, pseudopodia are extended around the organism, encasing it in a phagocytic vacuole which becomes lined by the invaginated cell membrane. After the offending organism is sequestered in the phagocytic vacuole, an integrated series of morphologic and metabolic changes occur, converting the phagocytic vacuole into a "microbicidal trap."

Mature granulocytes and monocytes contain at least two distinct populations of cytoplasmic granules which contain a variety of hydrolytic, digestive, and antimicrobial proteins and enzymes.[12] In the process of degranulation these granules approach and fuse with the membrane of the phagocytic vacuole, discharging their contents in contained proximity to the sequestered organisms (Figure 4).

Coincident with phagocytosis there is also a major increase in oxidative metabolism, the so-called "respiratory burst" of phagocytosis. The major metabolic features of the respiratory burst are marked increases in oxygen consumption, the production of hydrogen peroxide (H_2O_2) and superoxide (O_2^-), and glucose oxidation via the hexose monophosphate shunt.[13] As shown in Figure 5, the critical enzyme is an NADPH-linked, cyanide-resistant oxidase (primary oxidase) which reduces oxygen to superoxide. Superoxide then combines with two hydrogen ions (the dismutation reaction) to form hydrogen peroxide, and the glutathione cycle scavenges any intracellular H_2O_2, converting it to water.

The stimulus for activation of the hexose shunt is $NADP^+$, which is produced by both the primary oxidase and the glutathione cycle, and reduced to NADPH by the enzyme system of the shunt. Phagocytosis, therefore, activates a self-regenerating enzyme system which consumes oxygen and produces H_2O_2 and O_2^-. Both of these substances are highly reactive oxidizing agents and either directly or indirectly produce potent antimicrobial activity.[14] The rare human genetic leukocyte disorder *chronic granulomatous disease* (CGD) illustrates the clinical importance of this oxidase system as a microbicidal mechanism. Leukocytes from patients with the CGD syndrome phagocytize organisms normally, but activation of the respiratory burst does not occur and a variety of common bacteria and fungi are resistant to these leukocytes.[15] Clinically, the CGD patients are profoundly susceptible to infection—especially by *Staphylococcus aureus*, *Escherichia coli*,

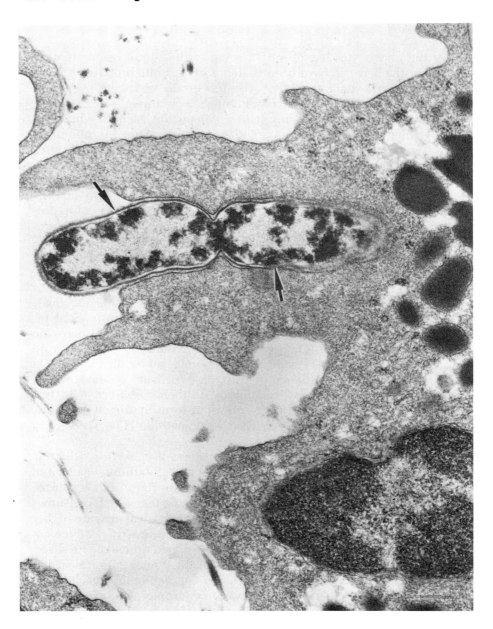

FIG. 3.   Phagocytosis of E. coli by a polymorphonuclear leukocyte. Pseudo-podia are extended around the bacteria, encasing them in a phagocytic vacuole which is lined by invaginated cell membrane. (Electron micrograph courtesy of Dr. Dorothy Bainton.)

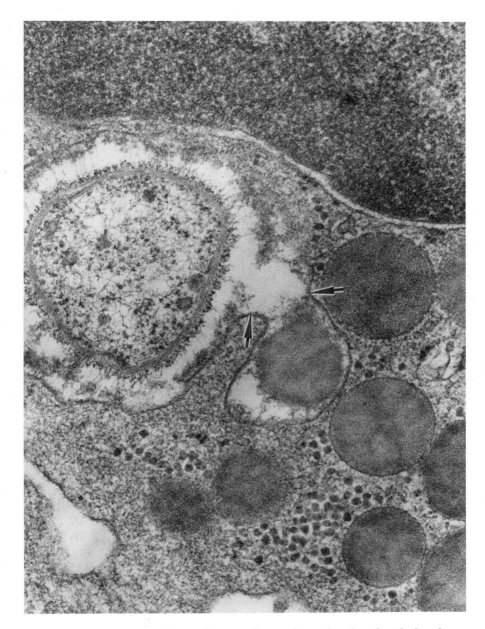

FIG. 4.   During degranulation the granule membrane has fused with the phagocytic vacuole, exposing the ingested bacterium to the granule enzymes. (Electron micrograph courtesy of Dr. Dorothy Bainton.)

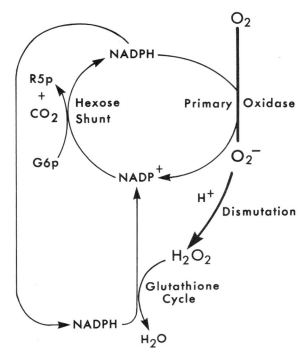

Fig. 5. The NADPH-linked primary oxidase reduces oxygen to superoxide radical (O_2^-). Enzymatic or spontaneous dismutation of superoxide produces hydrogen peroxide, an important microbicidal agent. $NADP^+$ is also produced by the glutathione cycle, which may protect the cell from excess levels of hydrogen peroxide, and NADPH is regenerated by the hexose shunt.

Pseudomonas, Salmonella, Serratia, and a variety of gram-negative organisms of low pathogenicity. Many of these organisms can also cause infection in surgical wounds. The biochemical details of how degranulation and the respiratory burst lead to microbial killing have been greatly elucidated in the past five years and deserve further examination.

LEUKOCYTE MICROBICIDAL MECHANISMS

Killing mechanisms of the leukocyte can be grouped into two categories: those that depend on oxygen for generation of microbicidal agents and those such as degranulation that function equally well in the absence of oxygen.

Oxygen-Dependent Microbicidal Mechanisms

The most extensively studied mechanism of oxygen-dependent microbial killing is mediated by myeloperoxidase, which is present in the
primary granules of neutrophils and monocytes. In the presence of
small amounts of H_2O_2 and halide ions (I^-, Cl^-, or Br^-), a potent microbicidal system of broad specificity is formed.[16] Myeloperoxidase
(MPO) catalyzes the oxidation of halide ions (X^-) to hypohalite ions
by H_2O_2.

$$X^- + H_2O_2 \xrightarrow{\text{MPO}} XO^- + H_2O$$

The precise killing mechanisms of this system are controversial. One
of the consequences of the above reaction is that halide ions are incorporated into the bacterial cell wall, but the correlation between halide incorporation and bacterial killing is weak. Second, the myeloperoxidase system converts carboxyl groups of bacterial cell wall amino
acids to aldehydes and this, in some way, may result in bacterial killing. The myeloperoxidase-mediated system may also form singlet oxygen, another highly reactive oxygen species which, in turn, may kill
organisms by the disruption of double bonds in the structure of the
microbial wall.[14]

Several patients with myeloperoxidase deficiency have been identified and the killing of bacteria and fungi by their leukocytes is somewhat delayed.[17] In contrast to patients with the CGD syndrome whose
leukocytes do not generate toxic oxygen moieties, the myeloperoxi-
dase-deficient patients show little clinical susceptibility to infection.
It is evident that oxygen derivatives must mediate bacterial killings by
mechanisms that do not require myeloperoxidase mediation. In relatively high concentrations (e.g., 0.5 mM) hydrogen peroxide is directly
toxic to certain organisms, and the sensitivity of an organism to H_2O_2
depends on its content of catalase, which degrades H_2O_2.[18] Certain
other organisms liberate H_2O_2 and thus contribute to their own death
in the confines of the phagocytic vacuole. Such "kamikaze" bacteria
are also effectively killed by CGD neutrophils because H_2O_2 produced
by the organism substitutes for the defective H_2O_2 production of CGD
leukocytes.[19]

In a similar manner, superoxide may directly kill certain organisms,
although the evidence for this is somewhat less secure.[14] The sensitivity of an organism to O_2^- may depend on its content of superoxide
dismutase (SOD), an enzyme that degrades superoxide. There appears
to be a general correlation between the air tolerance of an organism

and its content of SOD: anaerobes have little or no SOD whereas aerobes have high levels of SOD.[20]

Emerging evidence suggests that phagocytizing leukocytes also generate hydroxyl radicals (OH·) and singlet oxygen (O_2^*) which are both highly unstable and highly reactive oxygen derivatives. Hydroxyl-radical-generating systems have been shown to kill bacteria avidly in vitro and indirect evidence that O_2^* is involved in killing of certain bacteria has also been provided.[14]

Although the specific microbicidal mechanisms are only partially understood, it is now evident that the oxygen/NADPH oxidase system of leukocytes contributes an extremely important but perhaps vulnerable antimicrobial defense mechanism (see Chapter 22).

Oxygen-Independent Systems

Evidence for oxygen-independent killing mechanisms is provided by two types of studies. First, leukocytes incubated in the absence of O_2 retain microbicidal capacity against certain microbes, while other organisms are protected by anoxia. Second, antimicrobial substances extracted from leukocytes are capable of killing some types of organisms in vitro in the absence of O_2.

Among these oxygen-independent agents are (1) acid, which is formed in the phagocytic vacuole and which can directly kill certain acid-sensitive organisms, (2) lactoferrin, which is present in leukocyte granules and exerts a microbistatic effect by the chelation of iron required for microbial growth, (3) lysozyme, an abundant leukocyte granule enzyme, which digests cell wall constituents and contributes to the killing and digestion of organisms, and (4) granule cationic proteins, which are a group of highly cationic proteins that bind to the surface of ingested organisms and mediate microbial killing.[16] Emerging evidence suggests that this latter system may be of major importance in the antimicrobial armament of the leukocyte.[21]

CLINICAL IMPORTANCE OF OXYGEN-DEPENDENT KILLING MECHANISMS

Figure 6 illustrates several important points about oxygen-dependent killing mechanisms. The generation of O_2^- and H_2O_2 from molecular oxygen is responsible for much of the antimicrobial capacity of normal phagocytes. In the CGD syndrome, deficiency of a functional oxidase enzyme system prevents the generation of O_2^- and H_2O_2 and, as a consequence, bacterial killing is greatly impaired and susceptibility to

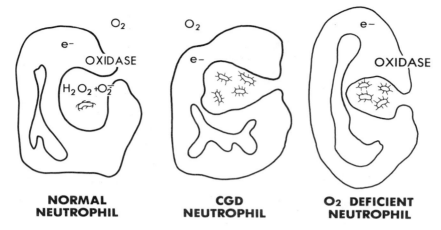

FIG. 6. *Normal neutrophils consume O_2, generate H_2O_2 and O_2^-, and kill bacteria effectively. CGD neutrophils are oxidase-deficient and killing of many species of bacteria is ineffective. Oxygen-deficient neutrophils have an intact oxidase system but do not generate H_2O_2 and O_2^-. Microbial killing by O_2-deficient neutrophils is also ineffective.*

clinical infection is high. We might hypothesize, then, that deficiency of molecular oxygen should cause a killing defect resembling that seen in the CGD syndrome. Since injured tissues, and particularly infected tissues, are hypoxic, and since phagocytes utilize O_2 in killing bacteria and fungi, oxygen deficiency in hypoxic tissues could force the phagocytes into a CGD-like state and thus limit the microbicidal capacity of wound leukocytes.

We have recently performed a series of studies that lend strong support to the above hypothesis. In these studies *in vitro* killing of various bacteria by normal leukocytes in an anoxic environment was compared with killing of the same organisms by CGD leukocytes. With every organism tested, the killing capacity of anoxic normal cells closely resembled that of CGD cells. We were also able to demonstrate that oxygen availability influences susceptibility to wound infection and the rate of bacterial clearance from experimental wounds in animals.[22] An example of this effect is shown in Figure 7. In these latter studies, staphylococci were injected into subcutaneous wound cylinders implanted in three groups of rabbits which were maintained in O_2-regulated environmental chambers. It can be seen that the clearance of bacteria is retarded in the hypoxic group.

Among the important emerging concepts in the biology of surgical infection is that oxygen is an essential substrate for the effective killing

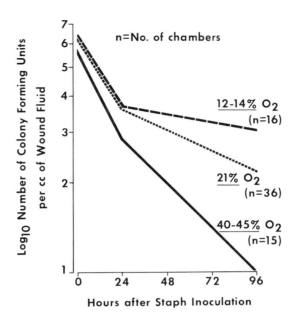

FIG. 7. *Staphylococci were injected into experimental wounds in three groups of animals, maintained under hypoxic, normoxic, or hyperoxic conditions. Clearance of bacteria from wound fluid was retarded in the hypoxic animals and accelerated in the hyperoxic group.*

of bacteria and fungi by phagocytic leukocytes. It also would appear that in hypoxic tissues small increments in oxygen supply may lead to relatively large differences in resistance to infection.

Microbicidal Competence of Wound Leukocytes

Most studies of leukocyte function have been performed using cells isolated from blood or from sterile peritoneal exudates in experimental animals. These studies are based on the assumption that such cells truly represent the cells that collect in the inflammatory site. The leukocytes that ultimately arrive in a wound, however, have been subjected to a series of events including margination on the vascular endothelium, migration from these vessels under chemotactic influence, and phagocytosis of foreign and cellular debris en route. For these reasons we have questioned whether such cells are injured or functionally altered in their journey to the wound.

In a study employing leukocytes recovered from small, relatively

**Table 1. Microbicidal Activity of Rabbit Blood
and Wound Leukocytes**

Source of Cells	Wound Age (days)	Reduction in concentration of S. aureus after incubation for 2 hr (%)
Wound	5	96
Wound	10	95
Wound	17	92
Blood	—	98

Note: Bacteria were incubated in the presence of rabbit blood and wound leukocytes and percent reduction in concentration was measured after 2 hours of incubation. (Bacterial concentrations were stable in the absence of leukocytes.)

atraumatic wounds in rabbits, both oxidative metabolic and microbicidal activities were found to be comparable to those of leukocytes recovered from rabbit blood (Table 1).[23] Furthermore, the functional integrity of wound leukocytes was well preserved during progressive maturation of the wound. Similar findings have been reported by Bell and associates, who utilized leukocytes recovered acutely from dermal abrasions in humans.[24] In that study, the phagocytic capacity, microbicidal activity, and the lysosomal enzyme contents of wound and blood leukocytes were nearly identical.

In addition to killing bacteria, wound leukocytes and macrophages also serve as scavengers that ingest injured cell particles, thereby internally debriding the injured area. The above-mentioned studies employed experimental wounds in which the amount of injured tissue was small. To assess leukocyte function in more extensive wounds, cells recovered from human radical mastectomy wounds were studied and the microbicidal activity was profoundly impaired (Table 2). Furthermore, the mastectomy wound leukocytes were engorged with fat

**Table 2. Microbicidal Activity of Human Blood
and Wound Leukocytes**

Source of cells	Change in Concentration of S. aureus After Incubation for 2 hours (%)
Blood	93↓
Wound	56↑

Note: Staphylococci were incubated in the presence of leukocytes from human blood and from human radical mastectomy wounds. Marked bacterial killing had occurred after 2 hours in the presence of blood leukocytes. A net increase in bacterial concentration occurred in the presence of leukocytes from wounds.

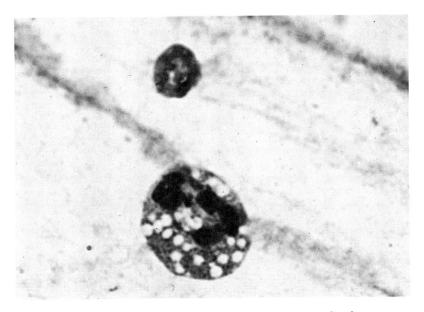

FIG. 8. *This is a typical neutrophil recovered from a radical mastectomy wound. Note the large quantities of ingested fat.*

and tissue debris (Fig. 8) which may have reduced further phagocytic activity. It is tempting to postulate that when tissue injury in a wound is extensive, leukocyte phagocytic reserves are expended in internal debridement with impairment of the capacity for subsequent phagocytosis and killing of microorganisms.

Antibacterial Factors in Wound Fluids

As we compared the functional characteristics of leukocytes from wounds and from blood, we also studied the humoral factors found in wound fluids and in blood.

Although leukocytes are required for efficient killing of most pathogenic organisms, certain gram-negative organisms are lysed directly by antibody and complement in blood serum.[25] Other blood proteins called β-lysins have been found to kill both gram-positive and gram-negative organisms independently of antibody and complement.[26] When bacteria invade tissues, they are bathed in interstitial lymph rather than blood serum. In a wound the interstitial fluid also contains products of tissue injury as well as substances released during the lysis of blood cells and blood clot. The humoral constituents in a fresh wound should resemble those of blood serum, while the composition of fluid from more mature wounds should resemble that of lymph. Martinez[27] has demonstrated that cell-free human thoracic duct lymph contains a variety of killing factors showing different specificities for various kinds of bacteria. Furthermore, these factors were not detectable in blood serum.

These observations prompted us to question the prevalent surgical aphorism that a wound seroma is an "ideal culture medium." All wounds, of course, are bathed in various quantities of wound fluid, and while most wounds are contaminated to some degree few become clinically infected. To test this, we incubated bacteria in fluids recovered from mastectomy wounds and compared microbial survival in these fluids and in blood serum. After four hours of incubation, wound fluid killed S. aureus and E. coli, while in blood serum the concentrations of both organisms were stable (Fig. 9). Two types of antimicrobial protein were identified; one resembled complement and was present only for the first three postoperative days, while the other was heat stable and was present in increasing concentrations as wound age increased. The growth of a number of other organisms was suppressed more by wound fluids than by blood serum.[28]

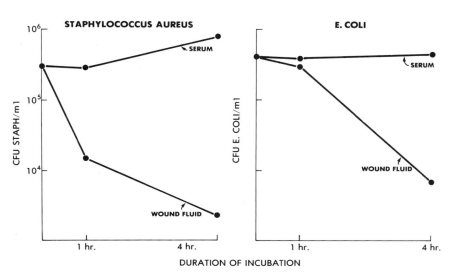

FIG. 9. Staphylococci and E. coli were incubated in human blood serum and wound fluid. Killing of both organisms had occurred after 4 hours of incubation in wound fluid.

SUMMARY

Surgical wounds possess a remarkable degree of natural resistance to infection. The microbicidal activity of wound leukocytes and the antibacterial proteins present in wound fluid undoubtedly contribute to their natural resistance.

REFERENCES

1. Ward PA: Leukotaxis and leukotactic disorders. Am J Pathol 77:520, 1974
2. Fernandez HN, Henson PM, Otani A, Hugli TE: Chemotactic response to human C3a and C5a anaphylotoxins. I. Evaluation of C3a and C5a leukocytes in-vitro and under simulated conditions. J Immunol 120:109, 1978
3. Hugli TE, Muller-Eberhard HJ: Anaphylatoxins: C3a and C5a. Adv Immnol 26:1, 1978
4. Fernandez HN, Hugli TE: Partial characterization of human C5a anaphylatoxin. I. Chemical disruption of the carbohydrate and polypeptide portions of human C5a. J Immunol 117:1688, 1976
5. Meakins JL, McLean APH, Kelly R, et al: Delayed hypersensitivity and neutrophil chemotaxis: Effect of trauma. J Trauma 18:240, 1978
6. Warden GD, Mason AD, Pruitt BR: Evaluation of leukocyte chemotaxis in vitro in thermally injured patients. Ann Surg 181:1001, 1975
7. Dionigli R, Zonta A, Dominioni L, et al: The effects of total parenteral nutrition on immunodepression due to malnutrition. Ann Surg 185:467, 1977
8. Alexander JW, McClellan MA, Ogle CK, Ogle JD: Consumptive opsonopathy: Possible pathogenesis in lethal and opportunistic infections. Ann Surg 184:672, 1976
9. Saba TM, Blumenstock FA, Scovill WA, Bernard H: Cryoprecipitate reversal of opsonic α_2-surface binding glycoprotein deficiency in sepic surgical and trauma patients. Science, 201:622, 1978
10. Macher AM, Bennett JE, Qadek JE, Frank MM: Complement depletion in cryptococcal sepsis. J Immunol 120:1686, 1978
11. Hahn-Pedersen J, Sovenson H, Kehlet H: Complement activation during surgical procedures. Surg Gynecol Obstet 146:66, 1978
12. Baggiolini M: The enzymes of the granules of polymorphonuclear leukocytes and their functions. Enzyme 13:132, 1972
13. Stossel TP: Phagocytosis. N Engl J Med 290:717, 774, 833, 1974
14. Babior BM: Oxygen-dependent microbicidal killing of phagocytes. N Engl J Med 298:659, 721, 1978
15. Hohn DC, Lehrer RI: NADPH Oxidase Deficiency in X-linked Chronic Granulomatous Disease. J Clin Invest 55:707, 1975
16. Klebanoff SJ: Antimicrobial mechanisms in neutrophilic polymorphonuclear leukocytes. Semin Hematol 12:117, 1975
17. Lehrer RI, Cline MJ: Leukocyte myeloperoxidase deficiency and disseminated Candidiasis; the role of myeloperoxidase in resistance to candida infection. J Clin Invest 48:1478, 1969

18. Mandell GL: Catalase, superoxide dismutase, and virulence of Staphyloccus aureus: In vitro and in vivo studies with emphasis on staphylococcal-leukocyte interaction. J Clin Invest 55:561, 1975

19. Kaplan EL, Laxdol T, Quie PG: Studies of polymorphonuclear leukocytes from patients with chronic granulomatous disease of childhood; bactericidal capacity for streptococci. Pediatrics 41:591, 1968

20. McCord JM, Keele BB Jr, Fridovich I: An enzyme-based theory of obligate anaerobiosis; the physiological function of superoxide dismutase. Proc Natl Acad Sci USA, 68:1024, 1971

21. Odeberg H, Olsson I: Antibacterial activity of cationic proteins from granulocytes. J Clin Invest 56:1118, 1975

22. Hohn DC, MacKay RD, Hunt TK: The effect of oxygen tension on the microbicidal function of leukocytes in wounds and in vitro. Surg Forum 27:18, 1976

23. Hohn DC, Ponce B, Burton RW, Hunt TK: Antimicrobial systems of the surgical wound. I. A comparison of oxidative metabolism and microbicidal capacity of phagocytes from wounds and from peripheral blood. Am J Surg 133:597, 1977

24. Bell ML, Clay RC, Howe CW, Rutenberg AM: Antibacterial properties of human inflammatory leukocytes: A comparison with leukocytes derived from peripheral blood. J Reticuloendothel Soc 11:167, 1972

25. Muschel LH: Serum bactericidal actions. Ann NY Acad Sci 88:1265, 1960

26. Johnson FB, Donaldson DM: Purification of staphylocidal β-lysin from rabbit serum. J Bacteriol 96:589, 1968

27. Martinez RJ: Bactericidal properties of human cell-free lymph. Infect Immun 13:768, 1976

28. Hohn DC, Granelli SG, Burton RW, Hunt TK: Antimicrobial systems of the surgical wound. II. Detection of antimicrobial protein in cell-free wound fluid. Am J Surg 133:601, 1977

Comment

The current thrust of our work in the laboratory is based on the importance of the behavior of the various cells of inflammation. We firmly believe that the major opportunity for surgeons to reduce the risk and magnitude of infection in surgical patients is to learn how to manipulate the capacity of white cells which deal with bacteria. A hundred years ago, the frontier was to recognize that bacteria caused disease; shortly thereafter, it was to reduce the number of contaminating bacteria. In the succeeding 80 years, the frontier has been to increase our technical skills in order to diminish the susceptibility of tissue to infection. In the last 15 years, the challenge has been to apply the principles of chemotherapy to the prevention of wound infection. Now, the major frontier is to maintain and increase the capacity of white cells to deal with bacteria.

It is fitting that the maintenance of blood volume and oxygenation is perhaps the first means we have of enhancing the antibacterial capacity of white cells. Some of the participants in this symposium believe that immunity-potentiating drugs such as levamisol will be the next. Perhaps we'll find that insulin will be belatedly recognized as an immune potentiator. The possibilities are immense, but it will be some time before the important alternatives are delineated.

Inflammation in Wounds: From "Laudable Pus" to Primary Repair and Beyond

22

Thomas K. Hunt and Betty Halliday

The major outward manifestations of inflammation in wounds—erythema, warmth, swelling, pain, discharge, "toxicity," fever, and necrosis—are frequently and prominently mentioned in surgical narratives from past centuries. Time after time, ancient surgeons describe the sequence of trauma, inflammation, infection, gangrene, delerium, and death. At least several centuries ago in Western culture, and—earlier in Asian culture—surgeons began to note that at about the stage of swelling, pain, fever, and discharge some patients hovered precariously and then retraced their steps toward well-being while others fell prey to invasive infection and died. One of the prominent means by which early surgeons learned to predict which patient would survive and which would die was to note the nature of the discharge from their wounds. In many narratives, the distinction was made between a watery brown discharge, often foul smelling, which characterized invasive, lethal infections, and "laudable pus," the thick discharge associated with localization of infection and abscess formation. Suppuration achieved its laudability because its appearance was so often followed by patient survival. We know now that with pus comes local inflammation and induration. For many years, surgeons felt that *any* therapy that induced local erythema early would tend to be rewarded with laudable pus and its sequelae of granulation tissue, epithelization, and subsequent repair. Erythema and pus, therefore, became a desirable goal of management! They heralded the assembly of host defenses and repair to "contain" the infection. This association of pus and repair was realistic for its time. It is, however, inappropriate today. In the nineteenth century, when the findings of Lister, Semmelweiss, and

Holmes, added to those of Pare, demonstrated that wound healing gives rather little outward evidence of its presence, centuries of usage collided with science; and the surgical world rocked with the echoes.

Ironically, especially for Lister and Semmelweiss, surgeons must always have known that primary repair could occur without infection. Hippocrates advocated primary closure in his youth, when he was physician to gladiators. Presumably, the sharp cuts of well-honed weapons were likely to heal primarily, especially when tended promptly. In his middle age, however, Hippocrates returned to the traditional (and in his day safer) methods of managing wounds by leaving them open. Every surgeon in history must have seen wounds heal primarily. By 1846 Fergusson, for example, accepted primary repair for incised and bleeding wounds, and recommended that sutures be removed by "eight and twenty hours."[1] At this time, fomentations to encourage suppuration were prescribed for wounds which were not selected for primary closure—the purpose, apparently, being to prevent "manifestation" of spreading inflammation. When Pasteur, Koch, Semmelweiss, Lister, Holmes, and Halstead had worked out their discoveries and had demonstrated with aseptic and antiseptic techniques that wound healing and the inflammation of infection were, in fact, *distinct and separable entities*, a major milestone in the development of surgery had been reached. At this point, with the addition of anesthesia and the discovery of the vascular system, the era of modern surgery began.

At about the same time, the clinical dimensions and complexities of the inflammatory process began to emerge. Metchnikoff discovered the phagocytic response to foreign bodies, and simultaneously demonstrated the initiating events of repair.[1A] Although no one realized it, the cellular response of injury and the beginning of repair had been seen.

By the early part of our century, surgeons accepted that granulocytes and macrophages could ingest and digest damaged tissue and bacteria and did so in wounds. For the first half of this century, these were the only roles ascribed to these cells. Probably, the first break in this inadequate understanding came when Savlov and Dunphy noted that wounds disrupted on the third day and immediately reclosed gained strength so rapidly that they reached normal strength—that is, the strength of the unopened control wounds—within seven days after disruption.[2] The same phenomenon was seen to a lesser degree in older wounds, and it could be largely prevented, but not eliminated, by excision of 5 mm of the wound edge, a dimension which we now know almost entirely encompasses the inflammation of injury. The full significance of this finding was not appreciated then and may not yet be. They suggested that a "wound hormone" might lead to cellular hyperplasia in the first few days after injury, and that this hyperplasia need not be repeated when the wound is reopened and immediately reclosed.

In the same paper, Savlov and Dunphy also observed that anti-inflammatory adrenocortical steroids suppressed repair but only when given at the time of the first wounding—not when given three days later. Others noted that use of adrenocorticosteroids was associated with a singular lack of inflammation, fibroplasia, and neovascularization. Sandburg and Carlson added a critical piece to the puzzle in 1964, when they confirmed and refined Savlov's and Dunphy's observation that adrenocortical steroids inhibited primary repair only when started before or immediately after injury so that inflammation was prevented.[3] They concluded that inflammation is an obligatory step in the sequence of the repair process. In other words, there had to be some property of inflammation which calls forth fibroblasts and the new vessels which supply them. This observation seemed to explain the Savlov and Dunphy observation, but left unanswered the question, What is that property?

INFLAMMATION AS A PART OF REPAIR

In the 1960s Stein and Levenson[4] and then Simpson and Ross,[5] Ross and Odland,[6] and Leibovich and Ross[7] began to dissect the inflammatory system with respect to wound healing. They soon showed that agranulocytopenia produced by specific bone marrow inhibitors did not impair primary wound healing. Of course, we know that infection will be more likely without granulocytes, but if infection is avoided, the rate of gain in tensile strength is normal. Lymphocytes were removed by antilymphocyte serum also without adverse effect on repair. This left the macrophage as the only remaining whole cell found in any number in normal wounds that could carry the message to continue repair. Leibovitch and Ross suppressed the appearance of macrophages in wounds with a combination of antimacrophage antibody and small doses of anti-inflammatory steroids, and repair suffered.[7] Soon after, Chvapil and Steinbronn achieved the same results with antilymphocyte globulin alone, though their report remains unpublished. The findings were the same in each case; fibroplasia, neovascularization, and rate of tensile strength gain (collagen deposition) were suppressed. Leibovitch and Ross had also shown that macrophages secrete a substance which stimulates fibroblast growth in culture[7] (also see Chapter 1).

Inflammation is inextricably linked to coagulation, and coagulation is also a process of extreme importance to response to injury and to repair. Dr. Ross and his colleagues soon found that the platelet, when stimulated by thrombin, produces a factor that stimulates the growth of fibroblasts. The polypeptide responsible for this effect has now been isolated and sequenced, and is called *platelet factor*.[8] Less well known is the fact that we have recently demonstrated that platelets and thrombin, as well as wound macrophages, stimulate both fibroplasia and angiogenesis *in vivo*.[9] We also found that macrophages accelerate fibroblast and vascular endothelial cell growth over 20-fold when the two cell types are cultured together. Wound extracellular fluid and culture medium in which macrophages have been grown stimulate growth of fibroblasts, smooth muscle, *and* vascular endothelial cells in culture as well.

In 1963 Heppleston and Styles activated cultured macrophages with silicate crystals and showed that the transfer of the medium to fibroblast cultures caused an increase in collagen formation.[10] Several investigators have shown that silicates stimulate intense fibrosis *in vivo*. Deigelman and Cohen have shown that when macrophages stimulated by *E. coli* endotoxin are added to skin (tissue) culture the tissue synthesized more collagen, but their work remains unpublished. Polverini and Cotran,[11] and Clark et al.[12] have shown that, while unstimulated macrophages from the peritoneal cavity stimulate no reaction when injected into the substance of the cornea, stimulated macrophages or those taken from wounds (in the same animal) will evoke not only a scar, but neovascularization and increased collagen synthesis as well. Granulocytes have no such function that we can detect. Evidence from our laboratory also indicates that macrophages may be stimulated by red cells and fibrin, but not by whole blood clot. Some endotoxins seem to stimulate as do zymosan and dextran.

The secretory product(s) of macrophages responsible for cellular hyperplasia have not yet been isolated. Opinion is divided as to whether they are hormones or enzymes. Several polypeptides from various sources that stimulate growth of fibroblasts and/or vascular endothelial cells in culture have been isolated. They include, among others; fibroblast growth factor (FGF) from the brain; somatomedin, platelet factor, thrombin, prostaglandin F2a, epidermal growth factor (EGF) from the salivary gland, and urogastrone (UG) from urine[13,14] The last two are similar molecules. Both inhibit gastric secretion. We recently surveyed FGF, EGF, and UG; all cause neovascularization when they are implanted in the cornea incorporated in an otherwise inert polymer.[15] Strangely, they produce little scar. Activated macrophages and platelets and thrombin produce both angiogenesis and scar in the cornea.

The implications of all these facts are clear. Macrophages are "activated" by substances found in wounds and can be further activated.

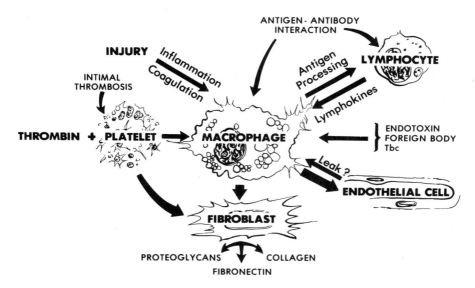

FIG. 1. *The current scheme of the cellular biology of wound healing. Note the central role that the macrophage probably plays. Apparently, the poly-morphonuclear leukocyte is reserved for defense against infection. There may be a lymphokine which directly stimulates fibroplasia.*

Although it has not been proved beyond doubt, it seems likely that after tissue injury, macrophages are first activated by ingesting necrotic tissue, red cells, fibrin, and possibly platelets (Fig. 1). More than this is necessary, however, to explain why wounds continue to heal after all necrotic tissue is gone. Perhaps the "activator" of macrophages then becomes fibrin which is found in wound spaces until they are totally obliterated. This, too, however, is not yet proved.

Some bacterial infections increase collagen deposition in the wound, but others seem to decrease it. As noted above, *E. coli* endotoxin, for instance, can stimulate macrophages which in turn can stimulate fibroblasts and vascular endothelial cells in cornea. In this case, massive scar results. On the other hand, if excessive numbers of granulocytes collect, they retard repair probably by consuming vital oxygen and other nutrients and by secreting collagenolytic enzymes. Some bacteria (clostridia, for example) secrete collagenases and "toxins" of varying noxiousness. This type of infection can literally "take over" and destroy the reparative effort. The following quote from Fergusson's *Practical Surgery*[1] is particularly interesting since he wrote it about 20 years before Lister's "discovery."

During several seasons in Edinburgh, some years ago, without any apparent cause, many sores in the hospital became affected with actions which, in some reports, resembled those of Hospital Gangrene. Healthy-looking ulcers suddenly lost their red colour, and became of an ashy hue,—the granulations having seemingly lost all vitality; then several patches sloughed, whilst ulceration extended and undermined the breach of surface.

CELL COMMUNICATIONS

Professor Silver (Chapter 2) further amplifies the above concepts and introduces a new idea that the spatial relations of the cells of reparative tissue are vital to their functions. His light and electron microscopic views of the tissue that grows into rabbit ear chamber wounds clearly show that macrophages are in the van, at the leading edge of the wound. Just inside are "immature" fibroblasts which secrete a gel of collagen. Within this gel, capillaries send out buds of endothelial cells to form new capillaries. These "buds" form arcs of new vessels in the collagen gel leaving the immature fibroblasts behind to mature and form fibrous scar collagen (see Chapter 10). This arrangement persists as the new tissue grows across the ear chamber and until it fuses with tissue from the other side at which time monocytes and active fibroblasts begin to disappear, and the vascular system matures into fewer, larger vessels.

These findings indicate that macrophages have a capacity to "sense" the wound space, or some chemical constituent of it and that in response they release a signal or signals which not only incite cells to divide but dictate the direction and probably the rate of growth as well.

We know a little about the signals that affect the direction of growth and the amount of collagen synthesis. For instance, Thakral has shown that placing autologous, activated macrophages into the dead space of a rabbit ear chamber 2 days after it is implanted hastens the appearance of new vessels by several days.[16]

Also, the wound architecture is partly governed by the energy needs of the wound (see Chapter 5). New vessels are constantly stimulated to enter the ischemic, acidotic, hypoxic area at the edge of the wound. Lactate levels are extremely high in this area, and investigation has shown that high lactate stimulates collagen synthesis in cell culture.[17] It is attractive to speculate that the lactate-producing macrophages (and the hypoxic fibroblasts) supply a lactate stimulus as well as growth and trophic factors and that these factors diffuse back towards the nearby regenerating vascular supply. When the pure growth factors alone are placed in the cornea, cell hyperplasia occurs but little scar results. Again, we can speculate that inflammatory cells produce the local acidosis that stimulates collagen synthesis. There is probably a delicate symbiotic relationship between new vessels, collagen, and fibroblasts. The new vessel needs collagenous support or it will burst. Yet the fibroblast needs the nutrition supplied by the new vessel in order to make the collagen. The symbiosis of the inflammatory cells, the new vessels, and the fibroblast—all in their characteristic spatial relationships—can be regarded as an interrelated "module" of reparative tissue, a delicate ecosystem which is upset easily.

Now that wound structure is outlined, it should be easier to intercept, stimulate, or suppress cellular signals. For instance, the addition of a small amount of endotoxin or killed fungus (both macrophage stimulators) accelerates new tissue synthesis in dead-space wounds. Timely injection of anti-inflammatory steroids suppresses secretion of macrophage factors and slows new tissue synthesis, while vitamin A restores monocytic inflammation and restores new tissue synthesis to normal despite continuing corticoid therapy. Although the "factors" have not yet been isolated, we find (as noted above) that the extracellular fluid of wounds is rich in growth-promoting material.[9]

CONTROL OF INFLAMMATION AND REPAIR

Metchnikoff classified wounds as "granulomas."[1] Unfortunately, "granuloma" became used to imply that the lesion had an infectious or chronic etiology; and wounds, of course, do not. From Metchnikoff's observations, however, interesting implications for wound healing arise. A granuloma consists of a localized inciting factor such as mycobacteria, fungus, silicate, or asbestos, some antigen-antibody interactions, some tumors, and perhaps other factors which are less well defined. All of these can excite a monocytic inflammatory response and, when they do, a localized fibrosis soon surrounds the area. This fibrosis is often a clinically severe and disabling problem. Data given here suggest that the problem might be treatable, but how would one do it? Ordinary medical instincts lead us to eradicate the inciting factor, the tubercle bacillus, for instance, in order to obviate need for the monocyte and allow the fibrosis to regress. Obviously, this is the preferred treatment of tuberculous scars. Bu what if we cannot identify or treat an inciting agent?

This dilemma pertains to hypertrophic scar. Histologically, hypertrophic scar and keloid contain fairly classical granulomatous reactions. However, an inciting agent has not been identified in them. Is it possible that keloids are the result of infectious agents, perhaps viruses. Or are they reactions to a foreign body? On the other hand, are hypertrophic scars just excessive reactions to trauma? If so, there is no inciting agent to eradicate. Is it possible then to interfere pharmaco-logically with the macrophage so that its encounter with traumatized tissue might not result in the excessive release of substances which ultimately lead to excessive fibrosis? Or is it possible to interfere with the signal from the macrophage itself? Although even the direction in which the answers to these questions might be found is still in doubt, these new theories of repair obviously point out a number of specific places to look. Whereas previous attempts to modify repair have fo-cused on collagen synthesis, lysis, and cross-linking (with only modest success, so far), we now have specific stimuli and specific cells with specific responses to study and modify. Since anti-inflammatory ste-roids are the most potent activating agents yet identified, this seems a promising area for research.

On the other hand, this may be a harder road to follow than it ap-pears, as Dr. Jackson (Chapter 3) might point out. Along with the stim-uli that lead to scar come stimuli that lead to collagen lysis. To control scar formation, the suppression of synthesis without the suppression of lysis might be like trying to balance a bank account with control only of deposits. Perhaps our new understanding of wound architec-ture might allow us the prospect of controlling these two aspects in-dependently—or, as we may wish, together. For instance, as Dr. Chva-pil points out (Chapter 11), colchicine seems to increase the lysis of wound collagen, presumably by specifically activating this process in leukocytes. It also increased collagen synthesis in their hands. The lytic effect was somewhat greater, and this drug holds some promise of therapeutic use.[18]

INFLAMMATION AS A DEFENSE AGAINST INFECTION

The second major concept of the function of inflammatory cells is to provide resistance to infection. All the major inflammatory cells parti-cipate.

Lymphocytes enter wounds, and once in position they are prepared to intercept antigens that enter the wound and initiate or restimulate antibody formation. Humoral antibody or cellular immune responses, however, probably play a relatively small role in the resistance to in-fection of primarily healing wounds compared with the less specific function of the granulocyte. Many of us feel that cellular immune pro-cesses are important in healing, but the evidence involving lympho-cytes in repair is scant.

Dr. Hohn (Chapter 21) has developed the outlines of granulocyte function. Probably all are operative in wounds. At first, the nonspecific or "natural" mechanisms of opsonization, phagocytosis, and intracellular killing are probably dominant. When wounds remain open longer, as in burns, however, the vastly increased, repeated exposure to pathogens must place increased responsibility for defense on acquired or specific immune mechanisms.

It seems that the reason why the wound-infecting pathogens are such an exclusive group has as much to do with the innate effectiveness of the granulocyte bacterial killing mechanisms of lysozyme, granular cationic proteins, and so forth as it does with bacterial "pathogenicity." Perhaps a weakness of this "natural" immunity "selects" the wound infectors that we surgeons so often culture from wounds. One weakness in the leukocyte seems obvious. It lies in the fact that leukocytes need oxygen to kill certain important bacteria that commonly infest wounds. All common wound infectors survive better in hypoxic tissue. The severe hypoxia of the wound space has been discussed in this symposium by both Silver (Chapter 2) and Niinikoski (Chapter 5). As Dr. Hohn (Chapter 22) has shown, one mechanism by which granulocytes kill bacteria depends on the presence of molecular (air-derived) oxygen. The schema for it is shown in his Figure 6. As he explained, one impetus for the discovery of this mechanism came from the rare, heritable disorder *chronic granulomatous disease*, or CGD, in which the severe predeliction to infection is related to the absence of an enzyme that converts oxygen to superoxide at the granulocyte membrane. Obviously, the absence of the substrate (oxygen) is equivalent to the absence of the enzyme, and our data literally prove that anoxic granulocytes have exactly the same degree of defect as cells from children with CGD. Thus, granulocytes which fall into the hypoxic wound space "acquire" a degree of CGD. Predictably, the bacteria that are not killed by CGD cells and afflict children with the disease are common wound invaders, i.e., *Staphylococcus aureus*, Streptococcus, *E. coli*, Pseudomonas, or Klebsiella. The remaining major wound invaders are Clostridia, Bacteroides, and anaerobic Streptococci, all of which grow and produce toxins best in hypoxic environments. Since CGD is often a fatal disease, this one factor would seem to be an extremely strong reason why wounds are susceptible to infection! Since oxygen is so important to the white cell, neovascularization then becomes part of the defense against infection—especially against *invasive* infection.

There is still more evidence that the circulation and its oxygen supports the leukocyte. We developed it according to the classic methods of Miles et al.[19] We chose their methods because they have demonstrated so many clinically important aspects of leukocyte and inflammatory function. In brief, we injected 10^6 to 10^8 bacteria into the skin of guinea pigs with a pressure injector. Several types of staphylococci and E. coli were used. Immediately *after* injection, we placed randomly selected animals in air, 12 percent oxygen, and 40 percent oxygen. Figure 2 shows the results of one experiment. Clearly, hypoxia greatly favored the development of necrotic, infective lesions in the injection areas. More telling, however, are the results seen when newly injected animals are placed in hypoxic environments for 3 to 12 hours and then changed to hyperoxia. Clearly, even after 12 hours of exposure to hypoxia we can diminish the severity of the lesion with added oxygen. While antibiotics are effective for only 3 hours, that is, the *determi-*

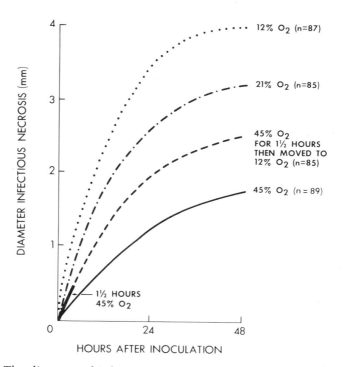

FIG. 2. The diameter of infectious necrosis following the intradermal injection of E. coli in guinea pigs. Note that the lesions in animals kept in 12 percent oxygen are more than twice as large as those developing in animals kept in 45 percent oxygen. Hidden in these data is an increasing number of lesions that never developed. In the 12 percent oxygen group, 60 percent of the lesions did not develop at all; in 45 percent oxygen 52 percent of the lesions never developed. The dashed line indicates that the even 1.5 hours of hypoxia can profoundly affect the fate of the lesion; this is consistent with the discussion of Burke in Chapter 19.

native period (see Chapter 19), oxygen aids (or hypoxia hinders) this response for much longer. This does not contradict the results of Burke; it merely redemonstrates the simple observation that while antibiotics may not penetrate the fibrin in the wound after 3 hours white cells do!

We have found also that the less oxygenated the wound, the greater the number of granulocytes that tend to enter it. Why this is so is not known, but the oxygenated leukocyte certainly seems a more efficient and capable cell. The surgical implications are obvious: gentle surgery with preservation of tissue and attention to tissue perfusion are the surgeon's major means of achieving healing without infection.

Wounds are also (often) acidotic to pH 7 or below. Some are hypercarbic to PCO_2 of 100 mg Hg or above. They are often (when hypoxic) also hypoglycemic to as low as 10 mg percent.[20] All these conditions might diminish the effectiveness of the cell, and none have been thoroughly investigated in that regard! Furthermore, there is dead and dying tissue about, which must be phagocytosed and removed. This consumes valuable leukocyte resources which otherwise could be directed against bacteria. Already, there is little wonder why the battle between health and infection is so often lost in a wound!

WHAT MAY LIE BEYOND?

We surgeons are absolutely dependent upon the ability of the human body to repair the damage we inflict during our therapeutic efforts. The scope of surgery over the centuries has been directly proportional to the degree to which we have been able to depend upon repair and resistance to infection.

Surgeons have always been proud of their results, but in our pride we have sometimes overlooked the need and even the opportunity for improvement. Everyone knows of Pare's bitter crusade against the then common practice of managing wounds by cauterizing them; his detractors pointed to their "excellent" results. Semmelweiss failed in his lifetime to convince others of the need for cleanliness. Though he dramatically reduced the incidence of puerperal fever to almost zero in a prospective "experiment," his detractors successfully (for several decades) cited their own results. Ironically, Semmelweiss died in a mental institution of "blood poisoning" originating in a laceration of his finger. When Lister had the effrontery to say that he could improve current therapy of compound fractures, his critics cited their own "excellent" results. He had the fortune to win his battle; though in the end, Halstead, Hutchison (with the steam sterilizer), and others rushed past him.

In the recent past, it was difficult to find a surgeon who could express discontent with the state of wound management. One fellow in our laboratory, who has contributed to this volume, was advised by his professor not to join us because "everything worthwhile knowing about wound healing had been discovered 50 years ago"! Recently, the ability of some surgeons to eliminate dehiscence and to lower infection rates in clean wounds into the 1 percent range, and those in heavily contaminated wounds into the 4 percent range, has attracted some attention, and hope for eliminating infection is rising. With the epidemic of trauma, disability due to scar and infection has become more common, and a desire to conquer it is being felt at least in editorial offices and granting agencies.

The question is, Where might our profession be if we eliminated infections, if we eliminated leaking intestinal suture lines, if we eliminated strictures of esophageal or biliary anastomoses, if we eliminated keloid, hypertrophic scar, and wound contracture? Pipe dreams? Perhaps, but 150 years ago it was a "pipe dream" to expect primary repair after *any* surgical procedure. Today we expect it and get it—*almost* always.

REFERENCES

1. Fergusson W: A System of Practical Surgery, 2d ed. London, Churchill, 1846
1A. Metchnikoff E: Immunity in Infective Diseases, Binnie FG (trans). Cambridge University Press, London, 1905
2. Savlov ED, Dunphy JE: The healing of the disrupted and restructured wound. Surgery 36:362, 1954
3. Sandberg N: Time relationship between administration of cortisone and wound healing in rats. Acta Chir Scand 127:446, 1964
4. Stein JM, Levenson SM: Effect of the inflammatory reaction on subsequent wound healing. Surg Forum 17:484, 1966
5. Simpson DM, Ross R: The neutrophilic leukocyte in wound repair. J Clin Invest 51:2009, 1972
6. Leibovich SJ, Ross R: The role of the macrophage in wound repair. Am J Pathol 78:71, 1975
7. Leibovich SJ, Ross R: A macrophage-dependent factor that stimulates the proliferation of fibroblasts in vitro. Am J Pathol 84:501, 1976
8. Antoniades H, Scher CD: Radioimmunoassay of a human serum growth factor for BALB/c 3T3 cells: Derivation from platelets. Proc Natl Acad Sci, USA 74:1973, 1977
9. Greenburg G, Hunt TK: The proliferative response in vitro of vascular endothelial and smooth muscle cells exposed to wound fluids and macrophages. J Cell Physiol 97:353, 1978
10. Heppleston AG, Styles JA: Activity of a macrophage factor in collagen formation by silica. Nature 214:521, 1967

11. Polverini PJ, Cotran RS, Gimbrone MA, Unanue ER: Activated macrophages induce vascular proliferation. Nature 269:804, 1977
12. Clark RA, Stone RD, Leung DYK, Silver I, Hohn DC, Hunt TK: Role of macrophages in wound healing Surg Forum 27:16, 1976
13. Ristow H-J, Holley RW, Messmer TO: Regulation of growth of fibroblasts. J Invest Dermatol 71:18, 1978
14. Ben Ezra D: Neovascularogenic ability of prostaglandins, growth factors, and synthetic chemattractants. Am J Ophthalmol 86:455, 1978
15. Gospodarowicz D, Bialecki H, Thakral KK: The angiogenic activity of the fibroblast and epidermal growth factors. Exp Eye Res 28:501, 1979
16. Thakral KK, Goodson WH III, Hunt TK: Stimulation of wound blood vessel growth by wound macrophages. J Surg Res 26:430, 1979
17. Hunt TK, Conolly WB, Aronson SB, Goldstein P: Anaerobic metabolism and wound healing: An hypothesis for the initiation and cessation of collagen synthesis in wounds. Am J Surg 135:328, 1978
18. Morton D Jr, Steinbronn K, Lato M, Chvapil M, Peacock EE Jr: Effect of colchicine on wound healing in rats. Surg Forum 25:47, 1974
19. Miles AA, Miles EM, Burke JF: The value and duration of defense reactions of the skin to the primary lodgement of bacteria. Br J Exp Pathol 38:79, 1957
20. Silver IA: Personal communication

Index

A

Abdominal adhesions, 135
Abscess, 188
Absorbability, 196–99, 203, 214–15, 217
Acanthosis, 83
Acid mucopolysaccharides, 2, 45
Acid production, 272
Acidosis, 287
ACTH, 145
Active sulfates, 50
Adenosine diphosphate (ADP), 60–61, 63–64
Adenosine monophosphate (AMP), 60, 63
Adenosine triphosphate (ATP), 3, 61–62, 64
Adhesive, 218, 222–23
Adipocytes, 108–9
Adrenalin ischemia, 244–46
Adrenocortical steroids, 283
Agar plates, 255–56
Age, advanced, 189, 192
Air, in operating room, 255–57, 260
Aldehydes, 140–41, 271
Allografts, 82–84, 88–89, 91, 97
Amino acids, 33–36, 38–39, 42, 65, 71, 265, 271

Anabolic steroids, 99, 101
Anaerobic glycolysis, 108–9
Anaphylatoxins, 143, 265
Anastomoses, colon, 153–58, 160–71, 173–80, 182–83, 184–90, 192–93, 202–3, 292
Anemia, 68, 189
Anesthesia, 243, 262, 282
Angiogenesis, 284
Antibiotics, 168, 170, 182, 199, 243, 245–46, 248–53, 290
Antibodies, 17, 25–26, 265–66, 276, 287
Anticollagens, 17, 25
Antifibroblast serum, 145–46
Antigens, 14, 29, 287
Antihistamines, 143
Anti-inflammatory drugs, 143–45, 282–83, 287
Antilymphocyte serum, 283
Antimacrophage serum, 145–46, 283
Antiseptics, 199, 256, 258–59
Antiserotonin drugs, 143
Aorta, 73–78
Aponeurosis, 194–95
Apoproteins, 73
Arginine residue, 265
Arterial wall, 72–74, 78
Arteries, 72–73, 107

Asbestos, 287
Ascorbic acid, 138–39
Aseptic techniques, 243, 254, 262–63
Atheromas, 77
Atheromata, 80
Atheromatous lesions, 72, 74–79
Atheromatous vessels, 31
Atherosclerosis, 72–80, 106–7
Attire, surgical, 258, 260

B

Bacteremia, 4
Bacterial infections. See Infection
Bacteroides, 289
Basophils, 4, 143
Biomembrane integrity. See Cell
  membranes
Blister formation, 81–89, 95
Blood cells. See Leukocytes; Platelets
Blood loss, 163, 192
Blood monocytes. See Monocytes
Blood pressure, 22, 25, 29, 68
Blood serum, 3, 6, 276–77
Blood supply, 56, 68–69, 71, 150, 185,
  189, 276–77. See also Leukocytes;
  Platetets
Blood vessels, 14, 29, 72–78, 106–7,
  202–3
Blood volume, 68–69
Bone, 42, 156
Bone marrow, 283
Bowel, 162–63, 180, 184–89, 202
"Burn index," 94–95
"Burn toxin," 238
Burns, 12, 14–15, 17, 25, 43, 81–95,
  97–98, 150, 266

C

Cadaver allografts, 82–84, 89
Cancer, 29, 190, 192
Capillaries, 2, 4, 16, 19–23, 25, 56, 59,
  64, 73, 93–94, 107, 151, 194, 204,
  264, 286

Capillary basement-membrane thick-
  ening (CBMT), 107, 110, 113
Carbohydrates, 46–49, 73
Carbon dioxide supply 20, 23, 59
Cartilage, 46
Catecholamines, 182
Cathepsins, 51
Cationic proteins, 272, 289
Cecostomies, 186
Cell communications, 286–87
Cell death, 144
Cell membranes, 136, 139–41, 147–48,
  151, 265, 267–69
Cell proliferation
  and atherosclerosis, 73
  and biochemistry of wound heal-
    ing, 32, 36
  and debridement, 239, 241
  and hormones, 100
  and oxygen and blood supply, 71
  and pharmacological aspects of
    wound healing, 143
  and physiology of wound healing,
    11–15, 19, 29, 31
  and sequence of wound healing, 1–
    10
Chalones, 14
Chelating agents, 137–138
Chemotaxis, 108, 143, 150, 264–66,
  274
Chemotherapy, 94–95, 156, 190, 192
Cholesterol, 72, 74
Chondroitin polymerases, 50
Chronic granulomatous disease, 267,
  271–73, 289
Cirrhotic lesions, 148
Clamps, 227
Clostridia, 289
Closure techniques. See Sutures; Tape
Clot formation, 10, 11–13, 19, 30, 277,
  284
Cloth tape, 218–19, 225
Coagulation, 1, 3, 10, 15
Colchicine, 139, 288
Colectomies, 155–156
Collagenases, 12, 40–41, 139–40, 153,
  157. 203, 285

Collagenolysis, 195, 285
Collagens, 1–4, 7, 10, 12–13, 15, 17, 20, 22, 25, 29, 31, 32–36, 38–40, 42–43, 51–52, 55, 57, 59, 66, 71, 73, 89, 99–101, 110–12, 118–34, 135–42, 150–51, 153–159, 163, 166–67, 170, 173, 175–77, 179, 183, 189, 194–95, 203, 284–85, 288
Colon repair
  collagenous equilibrium of, 153–59
  problems of, 160–83, 202–3, 215
  and unsuccessful anastomoses, 184–93
Colostomies, 157, 168, 186
Connective tissue formation. See Tissue formation, connective
Contraceptives, hormonal, 102, 145
Copper, 140, 151
Cornea, 284–86
Corticoids, 145, 287
Corticosteroids, 100–1, 145, 150–51, 189–90, 283
Cortisone, 100–2
Cosmetic results of repair, 208, 211–12
Cotton sutures, 214
Cotton swabs, 255–56, 262
Cytochalasin B, 139

D

Debridement, 145, 229–41
Degradation, 136–39
Degranulation, 267, 270
Dehiscence, 118, 160–63, 166–68, 170–71, 180, 184–86, 188–89, 201, 292
Dehydration, 12, 68, 81–86, 88, 95
Delerium, 281
Dermis, 81–95, 97–98
Devitalized tissue. See Debridement
Dextran, 284
Diabetes, 106–17, 190, 192
Disinfectants, 256, 258–59
Distal capillaries, 59, 64
DNA, 3, 6, 57, 100, 110, 145

Donor site healing, 89–93, 98
Drains, 186, 241
Drapes, wound, 255, 259, 262–63
Dura, 239
Dyes, 238
Dyskeratosis, 83

E

E + P treatment, 102
Elastic fibers, 2
Elastin, 32
Electrocoagulation methods, 95, 227
Electrolytes, 65
Endothelial cells, 12–14, 20, 25–26, 29, 151, 284–85
Endotoxins, 284, 287
Eosinophils, 4, 13, 143
Epithelial cells, 12–13, 15, 24–26, 81, 92, 97–98
Epithelial migration, 91–92, 94
Epithelization, 81–95, 97–98, 101, 225, 281
Erythema, 281
Esophageal strictures, 135, 140, 292
Esterified cholesterol, 72, 74
Estrogen, 102, 105, 145
Ethistrips, 218
Extensibility, 118

F

Face masks, 258
Fallout rate, 256–57, 260
Fascial wounds and repair, 201, 203, 226, 239
Fats and fat cells, 72–73, 77, 86, 100, 110, 147, 231–32, 235, 237, 241, 275–76
Fatty lesions, 72, 74–79
Fatty streaks, 73, 78–79
Female sex hormones, 102, 105
Fibrils, 39–40, 52, 121, 125, 157–58, 210
Fibrin, 226, 285, 291

Fibrinogens, 38
Fibroblasts, 2–7, 12–14, 19–20, 22, 24–26, 29, 31, 32, 59, 73, 80, 99, 101–2, 108–11, 113, 135, 139, 145–46, 151, 153–54, 194, 283–84, 286–87
Fibroplasia. See Tissue formation, connective
Fibrosis. See Wound healing
Fibrotic lesions, 135, 148
Fluorescein dye, 238
Forceps, 255
Fungal infections, 264, 267, 274, 287. See also Infection

G

Galactose, 36, 39, 50
Gangrene, 281
Garments, surgical 258, 260
Gauze, 225, 238
Genetic errors, 51
Genetic polymorphism, 33, 35
Globulin, 266
Gloves, 255–58, 260
Glucocorticoids, 100–2, 105
Glucose, 36, 39, 64–65, 71, 108–13
Glycogen granules, 12, 24
Glycolysis, anaerobic, 108–9
Glycoprotein links, 48–49
Glycoproteins, 32, 39, 266
Glycosaminoglycuronoglycans. See Proteoglycans
Glycosyl transferases, 50
Glycosylation, 36–37, 135–37
Gowns, surgical, 258
Grafts, 82–84, 86, 88–89, 91, 97, 239
Granulation tissue, 12–13, 15–16, 18, 39, 57, 89, 99, 101–2, 145–46, 194, 281
Granulocytes, 2, 9, 101, 267, 282–85, 288–89
Granulomatous disease, chronic, 267, 271–73, 287, 289
Granulomas, 287
Ground substances, 45–55
"Growth factors," 3, 287

H

Heart, 73–78, 203
Hematoma formation, 185
Hemolytic pathway, 265–66
Hemorrhage (shock), 1, 11, 22–23, 25, 68, 82, 182, 189
Hemostats, 255
Hepatocytes, 108
Homeostasis, 143
Homografts, 82
Hormones, 13, 99–102, 105, 145, 282–84
Host resistance. See Resistance, host
Humidity, in operating room, 256
Hydrogen peroxide production, 267, 271
Hydroxylation, 36–37, 135–37
Hyperalimentation, 171, 180, 192
Hyperbaric oxygen, 93–94, 97–98
Hyperglycemia, 106, 108, 110, 112–13
Hyperoxemia, 59–60
Hyperoxia, 57, 64, 289–91
Hyperplasia, 282–283, 286
Hypertension, 72, 107
Hypertrophic scars, 43, 135, 148, 151, 287–88, 292
Hypoglycemia, 291
Hypoproteinemia, 162, 171, 173–80
Hypotension, 189
Hypothalmic factors, 105
Hypovolemia, 19, 21–22, 25, 30, 68, 156, 163, 183, 189
Hypoxemia, 60, 189
Hypoxia, 22, 56–57, 64, 68, 80, 107, 156, 163, 241, 273
"Hypoxic" iso-enzymes, 73

I

Immunity-potentiating drugs, 280
Infection
    biology of, 214–28
    from burns, 82, 94
    and collagen morphology, 118

Infection (*cont.*)
  and colon repair, 154, 158, 163, 167–68, 170, 182–83, 185, 188–90, 192
  control in operating room, 254–63
  and debridement, 229–41
  and diabetes, 106, 108, 113–14
  host resistance to, 242–47, 249, 254, 263, 264–78, 280
  and oxygen and blood supply, 71
  physiology of, 242–53
  and physiology of wound healing, 12–13, 19, 23–24
  and sequence of wound healing, 2, 4–5
  and sutures and tape, 195, 199–203, 209, 211, 214–28
Inflammatory response
  from burns, 83
  and collagen lysis, 157
  of colon, 162–63
  and debridement, 230
  and diabetes, 108–11, 113–14, 117
  and hormones, 99–102
  and infection, 243, 247, 274, 280, 281–92
  and oxygen and blood supply, 56–57
  and pharmacological aspects of wound healing, 143–48, 150
  and physiology of wound healing, 19, 23
  and sequence of wound healing, 1–10
  and sutures and tape, 199, 208–9, 215
Ingestion, 265–67, 270
Instruments, in operating room, 255, 257, 260
Insulin, 99, 106, 108–13, 117, 280
Intraluminal pressure, 188, 203
Ionic concentrations, 14, 18–19, 23, 144, 271
Irrigation, high pressure, 239
Ischemia, 19, 56, 71, 113–14, 190, 244–46
Isolator drapes, 227

J

Joints, 150

K

Keloids, 39–41, 43, 135, 148, 287–88, 292
Keratan sulfate chains, 45–49, 51
Kidney failure, 190
Kidney transplants, 100, 106–7

L

Lactoferrin, 272
"Lag phase," 9
Laparotomies, 156
Lasers, 95
Lathyrism, 140
"Laudable pus," 281
Lesions, 72, 74–79, 135, 148, 244–47, 287, 290
Leukocytes, 1–2, 13, 71, 108–10, 112, 117, 143–45, 151, 153, 183, 230–32, 235, 238, 241, 264–65, 267–76, 278, 280, 285, 288–89, 291. *See also* Blood supply
Levamisol, 280
Linkage regions, 47–48
Lipid peroxidation, 147, 151
Lymph and lymph nodes, 14, 276–77
Lymphatics, 73
Lymphocytes, 5, 9, 13–14, 26, 283, 288
Lysis and synthesis, collagen, 153–59, 163, 189, 194–95, 286–88
Lysosomal enzymes, 3, 51, 143–44, 153, 275
Lysosomes, 51, 101, 147
Lysozyme, 272, 289

M

Macrophages, 2, 4–7, 9, 12–15, 19, 25–26, 29–30, 80, 101, 105, 109, 139, 143–47, 150, 183, 282–86, 288

Malnutrition. See Nutrient supply
Masks, face, 258
Mast cells, 143
Mastectomies, 66–68, 241, 275–77
Membranes. See Cell membranes
Mesenchyme cells, 13, 20
Mesenteric vessels, 185
Metabolism
  and atherosclerosis, 73, 78
  and burns, 95, 98
  cell, 99, 101
  collagen, 135–42, 167–68, 170, 183
  and diabetes, 108, 110–113
  oxidative, 267
  wound, 59–64, 129
Metabolites, 73
Microbial killing, 264, 270–277, 289
Microedema, 22
Microporous tape, 218, 220–223
Monocytes, 2, 4–6, 109–10, 264–65, 267, 271, 286
Monocytopenia, 6
Mononuclear phagocytes, 5–7
Mucopolysaccharides, 2, 45
Mucormycosis, 108
Muscle, 3–4, 31, 107, 231–32, 237–39, 284
Mycobacteria, 287
Myeloperoxidase, 271
Myofibrils, 12, 31

N

Neovascularization, 71, 79–80, 283–84, 289
Nerves, 238–39
Neutropenia, 4
Neutrophils, 2, 4–5, 23, 29, 264–66, 271, 273, 276
Nonwoven microporous tapes, 218, 220–23
Nutrient supply, 64–65, 69, 73, 107, 144–45, 171–80, 189, 266, 285
Nylon sutures, 214–15

O

Obesity, 107–8, 190

Operating room, infection control in, 254–63
Opsonins, 265–66
Opsonization, 264–66, 289
Osmolarity, 25
Oxidases, 267, 270–72
Oxidative metabolism, 267
Oxygen, hyperbaric, 93–94, 97–98
Oxygen-dependent microbial killing, 271–72
Oxygen-independent microbial killing, 272
Oxygen supply, 56–69, 71, 72–73, 107, 151, 189, 194, 274, 285, 290–91
Oxygen tension, 14, 18–20, 22–26, 31. 56, 58–59, 65–68, 73–78, 80
Oxygenation, 66–69, 151–52, 194, 204

P

Paper tape, 223
Pathological fibrosis, 118, 131
Patients, in operating room, 256, 258–60
Penicillin, 246
Percutaneous sutures, 215–17, 225, 227
Perfusion, 194, 204
Peritoneum, 182, 186
Peritonitis, 158, 167–68, 170, 183, 188
Peroxidation, lipid, 147, 151
Personnel, in operating room, 256, 258–60
pH concentrations, 14, 19, 21, 23–24, 26, 38
Phagocytosis and phagocytes, 6–7, 12, 19, 26, 101, 108, 143, 230–32, 235, 238, 264–69, 272–76, 289, 291
Phospholipids, 73
Pituitary hormones, 105
Plasma serum, 3, 6, 13
Platelet factor, 284
Platelets, 3–4, 7, 9–10, 13, 30, 143–44, 283–85. See also Blood supply
Pliability, 118
Poloxamer-iodine compounds, 259

Polyalkylacrylate adhesive, 218
Polyglycolic acid sutures, 215
Polymerization, 139–41
Polymorphonuclear leukocytes, 143–45, 285
Polymorphonuclear neutrophils, 2, 4, 12, 194
Polyonetholesulfonate (liquoid), 244
Polypeptide chains, 33, 35, 135, 284
Polypropylene sutures, 214–15
Porosity, 218
Prednisolone, 101
Pressure necrosis, 15
Preventive antibiotics, 250–53
Procollagens, 35–38, 42
Progeria, 110
Progesterone, 102, 105, 145
Proline analogs, 137–38
Properdin pathway, 265–266
Proteases, 153, 265
Protein polysaccharide complex, 45
Proteins, 45–52, 73, 100, 110, 120, 173–80, 256, 265, 267, 272, 276, 278, 289
Proteoglycans, 2, 13, 32, 45–55, 73, 135
Proteolytic enzymes, 95, 101
Protocollagens, 13, 25
Proximal diversion, 186
Puerperal fever, 291
Pulmonary failure, 151
Pus, 225–26, 228, 232, 248, 281

R

Radiation, 192
Rectum, 160, 162, 186–87
Red blood cells. See Platelets
Reepithelization, 93–94
Reinforced Steri-strips, 218
Renal failure, 190
Resistance, host, 242–247, 249, 254, 263, 264–78, 280
"Respiratory burst," 267, 270
Respiratory rate, 64
Resutured wounds, 201–2
Rete pegs, 15, 91

Reticuloendothelial system, 266
Rheumatoid arthritis, 29, 139, 147
RNA, 57, 110
Rodac plates, 255
Rupture, 118–19

S

Scab formation, 12, 24
Scar collagens, 38–43, 120, 129, 286
Scar formation
    and biochemistry of wound healing, 32, 38–43
    and collagen morphology, 118, 125, 128–31
    and collagens, 32, 38–43
    and inflammatory response, 284–87, 292
    and pharmacological aspects of wound healing, 135, 140, 146, 148, 151
    and physiological aspects of wound healing, 13, 15
    and proteoglycans, 52
    and sequence of wound healing, 2, 9
    and sutures and tape, 203, 210–11
Scirrhous breast cancer, 29
Secretion, 135–39, 285, 287
Septicemia, 4
Serositis, 189
Serotonin, 3, 143
Sex hormones, female, 102, 105
Shedding, microbial, 260
Shock. See Hemorrhage
Silicate, 287
Silk sutures, 214, 243
Skin, 81–98, 119, 156, 171, 203, 218, 222–23, 225, 227, 231–33, 235, 238, 241
"Skin flora," 258–59
Somatotropin, 99
Sponges, 255
Sterile conditions, 254–60
Steri-strips, 218
Steroids, 9, 99–101, 145, 150–51, 189–90, 193, 283, 287

Subcutaneous sutures, 217–18, 225, 227
Sulfates, active, 50
"Superhealing," 144
Superoxides, 150–51, 267, 271–72, 289
Surfaces, in operating room, 255–58
Sutures, 155, 157, 180, 185, 188, 194–204, 207, 208–13, 214–18, 225–28, 243, 292. See also Tape, surgical
Swabs, cotton, 255–56, 262
Synthesis. See Lysis and synthesis, collagen
Synthetic zones, 22

T

"Tackifier," 222
Tape, surgical, 199, 208–13, 214–28. See also Sutures
Temperature conditions, 38, 91
Tendons, 194, 238–39
Tensile strength, 32–33, 39–40, 56, 66, 100, 110, 118–28, 155, 163, 167, 173, 175, 209–10, 218, 283
Tension, oxygen. See Oxygen tension
Thrombin, 1, 3, 284
Thrombocytes, 3–4
Tissue formation, connective
and biochemistry of wound healing, 12–15, 29–30
and collagens, 32–35, 38, 42, 118–33
and debridement, 229–241
and diabetes, 110–11
and hormones, 99–100
and physiology of wound healing, 12–15, 29–30
and proteoglycans, 45–55
and sequence of wound healing, 1–10
and sutures and tape, 194–96, 201–2, 215
Tissues, 33–35, 238–239
Toxemia, 151

Toxins, 138–39, 238, 285
Transepidermal water loss, 224
Transplant wounds, 100, 106–7
Trauma, 25, 100, 151, 156, 162–70, 180, 182–83, 185, 188–89, 192, 237, 266, 281, 288
Trephones, 13
Triglycerides, 72
Tropocollagens, 35, 38, 42
Tuberculosis, 29, 108, 287
Tumors, 29, 162–63, 170, 287

U

Ultraviolet light, 257
Uremia, 193
Urethral strictures, 135
Urinary tract, 202–3

V

Vascular diseases. See Atherosclerosis
Vasculitis, 89
Vinblastin, 139
Viruses, 287–88
Vitamins, 65, 101, 147, 287

W

Weight, body, 100, 107–8, 139–41, 171, 180, 190
White blood cells. See Leukocytes
Wound cavities, 18–19
Wound contracture, 292
Wound drapes, 255, 259, 262–63
Wound edges, 19–22, 64, 68, 203–4, 212, 214, 223, 225, 239
Wound failure, 106
Wound healing
and atherosclerosis, 72–80
biochemical basis of, 32–44
and burns, 81–98
and collagen morphology, 118–34

Wound healing (cont.)
  collagens as biochemical basis of, 32–43
  and colon repair, 153–59, 160–83, 184–93
  and debridement, 229–41
  and diabetes, 106–17
  and effect of blood and oxygen supply, 56–71
  and hormones, 99–105
  of partial-thickness skin injuries, 81–98
  pharmacological factors affecting, 135–52
  physiology of, 11–31
  sequence of, 1–10
  and sutures, 194–207, 208–13
  and tape, 208–13

Wound infection. See Infection
Wound metabolism, 59–64, 129
"Wound risk," 207
Wound strength. See Tensile strength

X

Xenografts, 86
Xylose, 47, 50

Z

Zinc, 135, 140, 143–45, 147, 150–51
Zymogen, 41
Zymosan, 284